Pink Ribbon Stories:
A Celebration of Life

Tammy A. Miller

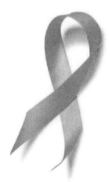

***Dear Lord,
Please use me this day
beyond my
wildest dreams!***

Pink Ribbon Stories:
A Celebration of Life

Tammy A. Miller

First Edition
ISBN 0-9701379-7-4
EAN 9780970137975

Tammy Speaks, LLC
Lighthearted Press
Copyright© Tammy A. Miller
All Rights Reserved
2011

Pink Ribbon Writers
Lacey Earnest, Kelsey Itak, Taryn Noll,
Kathy Salloum, and Diane Weller

Cover Photo and Design
Tiffany Dawn Earnest
www.tiffanydawndesigns.com

Pink Ribbon Editors
Ruth G. Miller, Linda Young,
Cynthia Finch, and Taliya Riesterer

For information, please contact:
Tammy A. Miller
E-mail: tammy@tammyspeaks.com
Web Site: www.tammyspeaks.com
(814) 360-4031

Check out all the latest information on
Pink Ribbon Stories
By scanning this QR Code with your Smartphone
OR
Go directly to:
www.tammyspeaks.com

Acknowledgments

This book has my name on the cover, but it is truly God's project. Thank you, Lord, for the wonderful blessings that have accompanied this entire project. Always keep me mindful of the many daily blessings and Proverbs 3:5-6 on this great adventure of life.

The book you are now holding is a true labor of love! Many people worked diligently to make this a reality. This section is to acknowledge their hard work and dedication to the project.

To the many women and men who took the time to include their stories within the pages of this book, I thank you! Without your willingness to share your time to create your stories and words to encourage, inspire and make us smile, this project would not have happened.

To the strong and lovely women in my life, especially my beautiful mother (my biggest cheerleader) and my incredible daughters, Tiffany and Lacey. I love you all so very much. You continually inspire me! I am very thankful for you being in my life every single day!

To the rest of my family for your endless loving support. Even if you're not quite sure what all this writing, travelling and speaking is about, you are always there to offer your endless love and help.

To my warm and wide circle of friends. You always help me find the humor, no matter what life throws at us. Friendship is a gift and you know I always tell people I am "gifted"! ☺

To Tiffany, Mary, Kimberly, and Dianne for all of your help on the cover, clean-up and details for the organization of this book.

To Lacey, Kelsey, Taryn, Diane and Kathy (and Tavrie!), also known as my Pink Ribbon Writers. Your assistance with this project was incredibly valuable. Thank you for your time to interview many of the people in this book and to write their stories. You helped people find their voices so they could encourage and inspire others.

To Ruth, Linda, Cynthia and Taliya also known as my Pink Ribbon Editors. You have spent countless hours scanning every word in this document to make it look as good as possible.

To the wonderful people at the Pennsylvania Breast Cancer Coalition (www.pabreastcancer.org). It has been an honor and pleasure to work with all of you. I am so delighted that this book can help to continue the fantastic programs you offer to help so many on a daily basis. And, well, you are just plain crazy – my kind of people!!

To Dr. B for saving my life. Even though you have moved onto another location and are no longer my active doctor, there will always be gratitude in my heart for being the head of my humor team! You saved my life so I can go on living, loving and laughing – thank you!

To the people who have made donations to offset the printing, publication and distribution of this book, no matter the amount of your donation. Without your generosity and support of this project, we would not have been able to move forward to help benefit many others. Thank you.

To Josten's for all of your assistance through the printing process. You made it much easier to turn the words on a page into a real live book! (www.jostens.com)

Dedication…

This book is dedicated to all the women (and men) who have
endured the challenges of breast cancer, or will at some point in
their life. We are from all walks of life, and each one has a special,
unique, story to tell.

For each story in this book, there are countless others from people
who inspire us daily through all that they do. To the people who
have come before us, and the people who will follow behind, this
book is dedicated to you with love.

Foreword
"PINK RIBBON STORIES"
Pat Halpin-Murphy

On this inspirational journey in life, I have been blessed to meet remarkable, uplifting women and families who have faced a breast cancer diagnosis with incredible strength, dignity and perseverance. From young mothers to prominent business leaders, politicians, grandmothers and beyond, I have true admiration for the countless women living with breast cancer, just like me, and those who sadly lost the battle. One such tireless advocate and dynamic breast cancer survivor who is a true friend and force of nature is Tammy Miller. Tammy's incredible zest for life has enabled others to gain healing power, knowing we all can fight to overcome the darkness that often is created by breast cancer. Tammy is a light in our lives. In *"Pink Ribbon Stories"*, Tammy shares the faces of breast cancer through a compilation of unique, insightful personal accounts of how cancer changes life and that as breast cancer survivors we do not walk alone.

Fighting cancer has been one of the most rewarding experiences in my life. Why? Over two decades ago, even though I was shocked with a Stage 3 diagnosis, was leading a fulfilling life as a Pennsylvania state official and mother of two college-age daughters, I quickly learned this major health issue would refocus my passion and calling. After barely escaping death twice from this devastating disease, I had a renewed sense of giving others the valuable gift of life. After a long, rough recovery, I plunged back in with immense enthusiasm. My stumbling blocks had become stepping stones. Thankfully, with the love and support from great family, friends and a fabulous medical team, I launched the Pennsylvania Breast Cancer Coalition in 1993 to educate, advocate, support and help others. Our goal is simple, "to find a cure now, so our daughters and granddaughters don't have to."

"Pink Ribbon Stories" offers hope and healing for those of us living with breast cancer. It is an exceptional resource guide filled with extraordinary spotlights on individuals and families. It certainly is a must-read for anyone who is fighting the disease or has a loved one afflicted. Thank you, Tammy, for this amazing and encouraging book. It underscores not to sweat the small stuff, that breast cancer isn't the end, to be grateful for each new day, count our blessings, lean on others, and NEVER give up! Yes, we all acquire strength in this journey, so make it count!

Pat Halpin-Murphy, breast cancer survivor
President & Founder
PA Breast Cancer Coalition

Reflections
Tammy A. Miller

Like many people in this book, my story as a survivor started when my doctor said the words we never want to hear, "Tammy, it is breast cancer".

Another one of my books, *The Lighter Side of Breast Cancer Recovery: Lessons Learned Along the Path to Healing*, details the entire journey so I won't try to duplicate it here. Instead, I will share a few words about my personal journey and some of the things I have learned as we walked through this incredible book project.

My Journey...

My personal journey began on September 14, 2001. I had noticed a change in my breast and we all know the saying, "if I only knew then what I know now!" I thought there was something different going on but when I went to the doctor and saw the physician's assistant, she wasn't concerned at all – the first thing – know your own body! Since it was close to the time for my mammogram anyway, I pushed her to have one done.

The experience was a familiar one to many people in this book. I get a mammogram and they call me back for more films because they "see something".

When I went back for the follow-up, the radiologist described what he saw and told me that even if he did a needle biopsy he wouldn't trust the results and he recommended I see a surgeon for a surgical biopsy.

Enter Dr. B! Dr. B is a man I had seen briefly a few years before, but I didn't know him very well. That was about to change! He turned out to be a wonderful doctor who became the head of my Humor Team (yes, clown noses, kazoos, and rubber chickens!) and was the man I credit with saving my life!

You may be wondering about the Humor Team and the other items listed, well, at the time I was a very active professional

15

clown known in my area as Hugz the Clown. As is the case with any well-stocked clown, I was armed with all of the above mentioned equipment, and a few other crazy things.

I firmly believe that we cannot always change what happens to us in life, but we can control how we respond to any given situation. I don't ever want people to think I am making fun of anyone with cancer, I am just choosing the best response I could, given the situation. For me, I knew I could not change the cancer diagnosis, no matter how hard I tried, but I had complete control over the attitude I brought to the healing process, and that was going to include humor.

There is a great deal of research indicating the positive, healthy effects of humor and a positive attitude in the healing process. The research isn't just for cancer but also for heart disease and other life challenges. In most cases, recovery is faster and better.

I had three surgeries along my path to healing and each one included clown noses, kazoo send-offs, and a few rubber chickens here and there. There were strange nipple send-of parties, with very interesting cakes (and strategically placed Hershey kisses), go ahead, use your imagination and you are probably right on!

I took notes of everything that was happening. I did this for a couple of reasons, first, I believe that when you are diagnosed with breast cancer, or any life threatening illness, you feel like your whole world is spinning out of control. You may feel that your body has betrayed you; I know I did, and writing everything down that was happening somehow made me feel like I had more control. I know, I didn't but the perception helped!

Some people journal their thoughts and feelings, and I was taking notes because I felt I could turn the situation into a book that might help others, much like this book will help others on their path to healing.

Throughout my journey I identified a few lessons that I learned along my path to healing. There were twenty in total, and I will share those lessons here:

Lesson One – Don't put off your yearly exams. Make the call – schedule the appointment.

Lesson Two – Trust your own instincts.

Lesson Three – Keep a record of everything that is happening.

Lesson Four – Develop a personal mantra to replace negative thoughts.

Lesson Five – Recruit your personal Humor Team! (No cost involved!)

Lesson Six – Be prepared to put up your own personal shield of protection.

Lesson Seven – Start and keep a "Recovery File".

Lesson Eight – Find love and laughter everywhere.

Lesson Nine –Tell your closest family and friends of your diagnosis in person.

Lesson Ten – Be informed!

Lesson Eleven – Remain positive in every single way that you can – no matter how small.

Lesson Twelve - Write down the questions that you want to ask.

Lesson Thirteen – Look for the smallest blessings in each day.

Lesson Fourteen – Know that you have choices.

Lesson Fifteen – Remember, you are a unique person!

Lesson Sixteen – Celebrate the smallest victories.

Lesson Seventeen – Accept that there are some things in life we cannot change.

Lesson Eighteen – Keep your doctors and health care providers accountable.

Lesson Nineteen – Thank your healthcare providers.

Lesson Twenty – Live life to the fullest!

*Except from: The **Lighter Side of Breast Cancer Recovery: Lessons Learned Along the Path to Healing** - Tammy A. Miller, Lighthearted Press*

There is so much happening when you are faced with this type of a health challenge and for me, identifying the lessons that I learned was very helpful as it made me feel like I had some control.

I believe all of these lessons are important, but a few especially stand out, like trusting your own instincts; finding the humor in every situation, remembering that you cannot always change what is happening; having a personal mantra (thought, prayer, saying, etc.) in your head because you can only have one thought at a time and **you get to choose** – you may as well make it positive; be informed; write down your questions; look for every blessing and remain positive; know that you DO have choices; and finally, live life to the fullest!

My life is truly blessed with wonderful family and friends and I am very thankful that I did not go through this alone. Above all, I know that none of us are truly alone, but we have the love of the mighty Lord to guide our steps – for me, I just need to remember to listen!

I truly cannot say that every day on my healing journey was grins and giggles, but I can say there was more laughter than tears, but it was my choice, as it is everyone's choice on how they will respond to any given situation in life. I pray that you will embrace every second of your life and that your path will always be blessed!

Thoughts on this book project…

For a few years I thought about doing a compilation book with stories from other people, but the time and topic just didn't seem right. That is until I heard Christine Allen talk about her story of keeping silent about her breast cancer for over 30 years for fear of losing her job in the 1970's (her story is in this book). I know that breast cancer has changed immensely over the years as far as detection, treatment, and recovery, but I sat there and listened and thought about how the mental part of a diagnosis has changed. Has it really changed? I don't think so. I am sure that anytime in history that a woman (or man) heard a breast cancer diagnosis; there was immediate fear and uncertainty. Yes, we do know now that the outlook is better than it was 30 years ago, and early detection, new medicines and procedures have helped immensely, but there is still a fear in many hearts and heads.

I sat there and started to think about how other things have changed over the years and that is when the idea of ***Pink Ribbon Stories: A Celebration of Life*** was born! A "celebration" you might ask? Did you notice that one of the lessons above was to celebrate the smallest victories (or ideas)? Okay, I admit it, I love to laugh and have a good time. Ready for a party to celebrate getting a new pair of shoes just call me!!

I was hopeful that I could get at least 50 women and men to share their stories as a survivor or caregiver or medical assistant. WOW!!! I never expected to have a completed book with over 120 stories!! In a small twist of faith – yes, faith, or maybe a little quirky, whenever I see a number that is in order like 234, or 456, etc., I always send up a little prayer of thanksgiving for the many blessings in my life. If you take the time to count the number of people who have a story featured here, there are… 123!!! Some days, I thought my e-mail was going to explode! I also firmly believe this may just be the first edition of a series, who knows!

There are all kinds of stories in this book. I am certain that something here will resonate with every reader. For some of the stories I should probably issue a "tissue warning", and for others a laughter warning, just Depends – yes, the pun IS intended!! There are stories that will warm your heart; make you laugh; cause you to pause for reflection; sometimes make you a bit angry; and others that simply tell a story of a courageous woman's journey through life.

I have noticed a few similar themes. Many of the stories share a faith in God, or other beliefs in the Power of the Universe. For some it is a renewed faith, for others a new found faith.

There are themes of the strength found in family and friends. How vitally important it is to surround yourself with people who care. There are a few reminders that we never have to go through this alone. If you don't relate to God or a higher power, we are also reminded that breast cancer affects many, many people, and there is always someone willing to reach out a hand of support – sometimes we just have to ask!

Another theme that emerged was a theme of thankfulness that cancer touched our lives, in fact some call it a gift. This may sound strange but there are many stories included that talk about a cancer diagnosis being the push needed to remind us of what and who are really important in our lives. In this hustle and bustle of life, which seems to get faster everyday, some people now look upon their lives in a different way because of cancer; a slower, more peaceful way.

Whichever story you find as your favorite, I pray that every person reading this book is touched by the stories and words that are written here to encourage, inspire, and make us smile!

For me, I pray that God blesses your path always and that your journey is somehow helped by a story or two in this book.

Thank you for the opportunity you have given me to collect these stories from these incredible people, and thank you for your support in reading along! May you always celebrate every moment, every detail of your life!

Blessings to you always and all ways!
Tammy

Author's Note: The next section of the book includes stories from those closest to me while I was traveling the journey to recovery. They include my mother, Ruth, my youngest daughter, Lacey, my dear "Pinky Swear" friend, Mary, and one of my best clown friends, Anita. From that point, the stories are alphabetical, but include some family connections, as noted in the stories. Read on and be blessed!!

I have also sprinkled a few "funnies" throughout the book. If you find a quote on a person's page, it does not necessarily reflect the opinion of that author...just a place to add some fun... ☺ For example, "Inside me lives a skinny woman crying to get out. But I can usually shut her up with cookies."-- Anonymous

From a Mom's/Nurse's Point of View
Ruth Miller

"Mom - I have breast cancer".

With those five words my world stood still as I was instantly transported over 40 years back to the time when I was a young nursing student. The dreaded "cancer" word was one that was only whispered among nursing personnel and NEVER mentioned in front of a patient. In fact, the diagnosis of cancer was not even listed anywhere on the patient chart. Diagnosis was listed in "code" as 31. The 3 was for the third letter of the alphabet – C, and the 1 was for the first letter of the alphabet – A. Thus, the 31 code informed all the medical personnel that the patient had cancer. Many times the patient did not even know! Many physicians were reluctant to even tell the patient she had cancer.

As a nursing student and later as a Registered Nurse, whenever I picked up a patient chart with the "31" diagnosis, a feeling of despair settled over me. I knew that patient was in for a long, debilitating surgery and for an even longer, painful recovery from surgery.

For twelve years of my nursing career I worked in the Recovery Room, which is now called the Post Anesthesia Recovery Room or PACU. I had the opportunity to see and talk to the patient before she, (almost all breast cancer patients were women then), was taken back to the operating room for surgery. I also had the responsibility of taking care of the same woman when she was wheeled into the Recovery Room.

When the patient was brought to the Recovery Room I knew her life had been changed forever! Her family members - husband, children, parents, and siblings were affected as well. They tiptoed into the room to visit and you could almost hear a pin dropped in the room – no one wanted to discuss that dreaded disease with the woman. Why, you might ask? At that time, a cancer diagnosis and surgery meant the woman usually did not survive past the golden window of "five years".

I remember looking at her chart prior to surgery and saw that she had signed consent to have a "frozen section" and a "radical mastectomy". This meant that while she was still under anesthesia a small section of tissue would be removed and examined under a microscope and if cancer cells were seen, both breasts would be removed along with part of the pectoral muscle, as well as the axillary lymph nodes. Even to this day, I do not believe she knew exactly what she was signing the consent for the surgeon to remove! Her first reaction once she was awake was to instinctively reach to see if her breast or breasts were there. The size of the dressings and bandages gave her some idea of what had happened while she was under anesthesia.

If she had a radical mastectomy her awareness, or perhaps it was denial, returned slowly. You could see the fear in her eyes and almost know the questions forming in her mind. "Now what is going to happen to me? How bad was the cancer? How long do I have to live? Will my husband still love me without my womanhood (breasts)? Will I still be pretty, sexy, normal?"

My job as a Recovery Room Nurse was to assure her, (even though I did not have the answers to those questions), that every woman was different and I felt that with the help of her family those concerns and questions would be answered in time.

Usually the day after surgery, and if time allowed, I would go to the room and visit the patient to see how she was doing. Many times when I entered the room, I found her sitting quietly, staring out the window. She was happy to see me, but I could see she had been crying. I felt so helpless! All I had to offer was an ear to listen, a hug and a promise to visit again the next day. After that, I tried to visit every day until she was discharged from the hospital.

For forty years I worked as a Registered Nurse. My duties were varied but I never forgot taking care of those women, from all walks of life and ages, who had this devastating disease called "Breast Cancer".

On Sept. 18, 2001, my daughter, Tammy was diagnosed with cancer of the breast. I was on one of my post retirement trips and when I called to check in with Tammy and tell her I had arrived at my brother's home in Arizona, she proceeded to tell me on the phone that she had just been diagnosed with breast cancer. She also proceeded to tell me that she had "hired" a Humor Team and I had been recruited to be on her Humor Team - IN THAT ORDER.

My first thought was "Oh, no. Not my beautiful daughter". Tammy is my only daughter and she is the light of my life. With my nursing/medical background, I knew the seriousness of a cancer diagnosis and what could happen to her. *I definitely did not see how any humor could possibly be found in this scenario - NO WAY. How could she possibly know that I would gladly change places with her on a moments notice!*

Tammy then proceeded to tell me that her belief was that, although she could not change the diagnosis, she could certainly change her reaction to the diagnosis. Her plan of action was to surround herself with only persons with a positive attitude, fun to be around, and with a sense of humor. There would be no time for negative thoughts about her surgery and recovery. Who better to fill that bill than a group of clowns?

Prior to her surgery date "Tammy's Team" had thrown her a humorous theme party with a "boob" cake, a size 44 DDD bra and, at that time, had presented her Humor Team with clown hats, kazoos, and clown noses. On the band of each hat, in bold letters were the words "TAMMY'S TEAM."

The morning of surgery arrived and Tammy has her hospital bag packed. No frilly gowns and girly stuff in her bag! Instead, in her bag she had packed a clown hat and nose for her doctor and well as a clown hat and nose for whomever assisted him during the surgical procedure. She also presented her anesthetist with a clown nose. In addition, she had packed two dozen or so clown noses to pass out to other hospital personnel who assisted in her surgery, such as lab technicians, nuclear medical technicians and recovery room nurses. Also packed in her hospital bag was a camera to record all the shenanigans for a book she planned to write titled ***"The Lighter Side of Breast Cancer Recovery".***

23

The time for surgery was drawing near and Tammy was transported to the surgical holding area. The anesthetist arrived and inserted an epidural catheter into her spinal area in preparation for epidural anesthesia. Two members of her family or team were allowed to wait with her in the holding area while waiting for the doctor to arrive. While we were sitting in the surgical waiting room, we began to see persons walking around the hallways with clown noses on. We knew that each one had done something to assist Tammy's surgical team.

The surgeon arrived and Tammy was wheeled back to surgery. I fought hard to hold back my tears at this point. I had seen this scenario so many times in my nursing career. Her "Humor Team" members were instructed to wait in the recovery waiting room until the procedure was finished. While sitting in that small room, we were each left to our own thoughts and prayers. I am uncertain what the other team members were thinking, but my own thoughts and prayers were, "Please, Dear God, don't let anything happen to my beautiful Tammy. She is so kind and generous to everyone around her. Please cradle her in Your hands today".

Tammy's surgery lasted approximately two and one half hours, although it seemed like an eternity. Finally the word came that Tammy was in the recovery room and that her doctor wanted to talk to us in a private conference room. My granddaughter, Lacey, and I sat silently in that small room for two or three minutes at most, not talking, just thinking - each one of us deep in our own thoughts. Finally, the surgeon arrived and gave us the good news. Tammy was now in the post-anesthesia recovery room and the surgery had gone well. He had performed a lumpectomy and had also removed five lymph nodes, which showed no cancer cells during the "frozen section" procedure of the surgery. Now, and only now could I let out a deep breath and enjoy being a part of Tammy's "Humor Team" - hats on, taking pictures, and playing the kazoo with the other clowns.

When Tammy awoke and showed us her incision, to our surprise, her surgeon had "bought into" her humor heals attitude and on the top half of her incision was a caricature of "Mickey Mouse", and under the incision was drawn a "smiley face".

Tammy's surgical recovery was unremarkable and if it were not for the bulging ice pack under her arm, no one would have known she had just undergone a major surgery. Of course, being the shop-a-holics that we both are, we had to go shopping just to prove a point! She refreshed the ice pack on her surgical site and we took off for Wal-Mart and the Mall to shop. The only difference I noticed in Tammy was that she kept reminding me that she could not keep up with my nurse's pace.

The only difference I noticed in myself was that I felt like I was walking on air. God is good! A Mom's prayers had been answered.

Ruth is a retired nurse living in Toledo, OH. She is the proud mother of Jim, Mike and Tammy (her favorite daughter – and both of her sons know it!); a loving grandmother of seven and a great grandmother of a one year old. She stays active in Toastmasters and enjoys cooking, reading, and travelling in her spare time.

My Mom
Lacey J. Earnest

It was October 2001; I was a senior in high school, and looking forward to spring break, prom, and graduating. It was an evening after school around mid October when my mom called me down to the living room for a talk. I wasn't sure what was going on but at 17 when your mom "wants to talk" I must have done something wrong. As I came down the step mom seemed very calm, I sat on the couch and I heard the words I never expected to hear out of my mom, "honey I have breast cancer". Hearing those five words I went totally numb, I couldn't think of anything but the anger that was quickly building in me. This is my mom she is not suppose to get sick, she is too young and has too much going for her. I stormed out of the house, mad that this was happening to my mom.

The next few days were filled with lots tears, and with the help of my very good friend Diane those tears were accepted and I was comforted with open arms. I didn't want to face this, in my mind it wasn't happening, but I had to face it and deal with it so I could be strong for my mom. I decided in the few days following the announcement that if my mom had to have chemo and lost her hair I was shaving my head. I didn't care about senior prom, graduation, or any other special event that I was going to do whatever I could to support my mom.

A few weeks later after the shock wore off, I was able to sit and talk with my mom, and she was completely open to whatever questions I had. She answered those questions to the best of her ability and the ones she didn't know she was very good about getting me the answers. The first big hurdle was I felt I needed to be home more to help with the house and just be there in case she needed me. I was able to leave school everyday around 10AM because I had all the classes I needed to graduate and there was a special program that I was accepted for that dealt with situations like this.

The next big hurdle was mom's first surgery, I don't like hospitals to begin with, and I really didn't like seeing my mom in one. My friend Diane made sure to be there with me, she never left my side. While we waited in the waiting room she would tell me jokes, we would laugh about good memories, and she was just a strong support for me. When the doctor came out and told us the news that everything was fine, and he was pretty sure he got it all I felt a huge relief, I almost felt like collapsing because this was the best case scenario. Seeing my mom in a hospital bed still groggy from the medicine was scary but the fear went away when I saw that the doctor drew a little Mickey Mouse on her incision site, and she was wearing clown shoes. I knew from that day on that my mom was going to be fine, she was going to fight this, and it would change our lives forever and for the better.

Going through the cancer with my mom made me stronger, because I saw how it made her stronger. She was given the freedom to write a book, and make her own decisions in her healthcare. She never had to go through chemo luckily; she researched and chose an alternate treatment plan. It has been almost ten years I have seen all the positive things that came out of her cancer, she had met some amazing people, she has been involved with organizations that touch so many, and most importantly she has showed me how important family is. I have always been proud of my mom, but now I am more proud than I have ever been. I have been told that I light up and glow when I talk about her. I see a lot of my mom in me, and I hope that I always have the strength that she showed going through this experience, and it is something I carry with me forever.

I LOVE YOU TAMMY MILLER and I AM SO PROUD OF YOU!!!!!!

Lacey lives in Port Matilda, PA with her big fat cat, Tyke. She works full time at Penn State University, where she is also a recent graduate. In her spare time she enjoys bowling, pet sitting and hanging out with friends and family.

The *"Pinky Swear"*
Mary Rogers

I do not think anyone is completely prepared for how they will react when their friend tells them they were just diagnosed with cancer. That happened to me on a day in September, 2001 when my good friend Tammy (author of this book) came back from an appointment and told me she had cancer. I was scared and wasn't sure if I knew how to support or help someone diagnosed with this disease.

Before I had much time to think about it, Tammy made me "pinky swear" that I would promise not to let her get depressed about it and would always stay positive. If you're not familiar with the age old tradition of "pinky swear", it comes from childhood game of locking pinky fingers and making a promise to each other about something really important. In childhood though, it was more along the lines of we wouldn't tell our parents that we kissed a boy behind a tree in second grade. But, this one was a whole lot more important than that and I wasn't sure if I was ready. I swore I would, but deep down I was scared that I wouldn't be able to keep my promise.

When dealing with Tammy it wasn't hard to keep my promise as she was more positive than anyone around her. It was easy for me to stay positive when wearing a clown nose and being in a kazoo band, or helping to organize a nipple send-off party. When around Tammy, everyone's spirits were always high. I was amazed, because here's Tammy the one going through all this and she was the real laughter leader. There were times that I was worried because I thought she was hiding her true feelings and eventually would crash…and crash hard.

I only saw a small glimmer of that once, Tammy called and said she was feeling a little down. It was after one of her surgeries and she was to stay in bed and rest, the weather was a little gloomy. Anyone who knows Tammy knows that she is always on the go and loves the sunshine. So bed-ridden and gloomy are not in her vocabulary. I showed up at her house with a ray of sunshine. It was a paper mache sun which was actually a piñata. I figured she could pretend the sun was out or take out her frustrations and beat it with a stick. That day was the first time I saw concern in Tammy's face. The topic that was bothering her was what she could eat. She was always a healthy eater and felt she took good care of her body and couldn't understand why something like this would happen to her. Since her cancer was estrogen receptor positive, and some foods create estrogen naturally, she was reading that she should stay away from certain foods that she considered healthy and was afraid to put anything in her mouth. In retrospect, we both think it had more to do with the hormonal changes in her body from her surgeries, as she broke down in tears, but at the time she was upset about what she should be doing. And, I wasn't sure what I should be doing either! This was the first time that I really questioned whether I was doing enough to support her. I guess because there weren't any clown noses, kazoos or boas. It was just me and a friend talking about feelings…real feelings. I was there with an ear and a shoulder to cry on and we made it through with smiles on our faces. But, it was after that day that I really questioned whether I was doing enough.

Fortunately, this incident was one of the very few times I witnessed Tammy without a smile on her face or doing some crazy antic, and I have since found out that there were a few grey times for Tammy during this journey but she never let them get her down. She made my pinky swear promise so easy to keep because she never let the grey times get the best of her. It wasn't me keeping her up and positive it was her keeping me up. I just had to be a good friend. There to listen, there to cry with, there to laugh with and someone always willing to go along with her crazy ideas. ☺

Tammy asked me what I would tell someone who just had a good friend diagnosed with cancer, or any type of serious illness. It is vitally important to just "be there" for someone, and sometimes that is to stand back for a little bit to see how a person is going to respond and what THEY need. Everyone deals with these situations differently, and by making yourself available to help with the smallest of tasks to the biggest, just being there to let them know you are there.

Tammy has a tendency to try and deal with all situations with humor. I know this isn't always the way people approach it, but I have found through reading the stories she has collected here, and the interviews she has done with people that it is important to view things with a positive attitude. Her platform when she speaks is that we can't always change what happens to us in life, but we can control how we respond. By going through this experience with her, I was able to see first-hand how the humor and positive attitude not only helped her, but helped those of us closest to her to help her get through an otherwise difficult and challenging time.

Being there for each other is one of the most important responsibilities of a friend and that can mean different things for different people, but just BE THERE. Oh, and don't be stingy with hugs, either!

Tammy has taught me that no matter what life throws at you, attack it with a positive attitude. It has been 10 years and I still feel like I haven't done enough and that she has helped me more than I have helped her. But, I will always be there to listen, to cry and to laugh with my best friend!

Mary lives in Bellefonte, PA and is the proud grandmother of sweet Isaiah, Hannah and Sophia. In her spare time, she enjoys spending time with her family, Kevin, Vanessa, Katie and Jeff. She is especially proud of her son, Kevin, as he serves in the United States Army. She also loves to have fun with her friends, which sometimes includes getting into trouble with her friend, Tammy, and is counting the days to retirement!

A Sprinkle of FUN from Tammy...

"When you're in jail, a good friend will be trying to bail you out. A best friend will be in the cell next to you saying, "Dang, that was fun".   --Unknown

Supporting Your Friend on Her Journey
Anita Thies

Authors Note: Anita is a dear friend who was right by my side during my cancer walk. She was the creator of Tammy's Team that my mother, Ruth Miller, referenced earlier, and was a wealth of assistance as she led the kazoo band and was responsible for a lot of the craziness associated with my recovery.

I asked her to write a few comments and suggestions that may be helpful for others in the role of supporter for their family and friends. Here are her words...

> Knock knock
> Who's there?
> Daryl
> Daryl who?
> "Daryl" never be another you.

"Daryl" also never be another friend quite like your friend, which makes supporting her journey a uniquely individual experience, both for her and for you.

Having been with friends who are courageous survivors and having had my own (different) type of cancer, I've discovered a few things that lighten the load. I offer them here for you to consider in your own caring outreach.

Presence and Presents

Your presence is the gift.

You may not know what to say and that's okay. You may be in shock at her diagnosis just like she is. Just be yourself. Say "I don't know what to say."

Words may fail you. Don't worry. A hug or hand squeeze will speak volumes.

Your friend will sense your caring because you called or came to see her, even if you felt inadequate for the situation. Stepping into the unknown calls forth courage.

You don't have to have answers. She doesn't have answers. Your gift is to be present to her in her time of uncertainty when she's had her bearings knocked out from under her.

Hope is Always in Season

It may sometimes be hard to be present with your friend in all seasons of her journey. It can be wrenching to see her fearful, hurting or despairing. In those times, it is tempting to try to "cheer her up" but often efforts to do so may leave her feeling more alone and isolated.

One way to be supportive without denying her feelings is to maintain an attitude of hope.

The late Eloise Cole, a friend who was nationally known as a bereavement specialist and clown, captured the role of the supportive friend in her widely shared poem "Borrowed Hope."

BORROWED HOPE

Lend me your hope for awhile.
I seem to have mislaid mine.
   Lost and hopeless feelings accompany me daily.
   Pain and confusion are my companions.
   I know not where to turn.
Looking ahead to the future times
does not bring forth images of renewed hope.
I see mirthless times, pain-filled days,
and more tragedy.

Lend me your hope for awhile,
I seem to have mislaid mine.

Hold my hand and hug me;
   listen to all my ramblings.
I need to unleash the pain and let it tumble out.
Recovery seems so far distant;
the road to healing a long and lonely one.
   Stand by me; offer me your presence.
   Your ears and your love
acknowledge my pain. It is so real and ever present.
I am overwhelmed with sad and conflicting thoughts.

Lend me your hope for awhile,
A time will come when I will heal
and I will lend my renewed hope to others.
---Eloise Cole, Scottsdale, Arizona

A Little Goes a Long Way

As you know, there are countless ways these days to
connect with your friend: In person. By phone--voice, text or
picture. Electronically--ecards, email, Facebook, Twitter. By postal
mail. By tangible gifts, remembering that the importance of
"presents" is that they remind her of your "presence" and the
loving support that surrounds her.
   You need not do big things. A little goes a long way. Some
examples:
   While I was waiting one week for test results, a friend
brought me a small wooden carving of a person praying, saying
she would be praying for me every day. I placed it on my bedroom
bureau. It was the first thing I saw in the morning and the last thing
I saw at night. Through the week, just the sight of it—reminding
me that I was being upheld in prayer--deepened my sense of peace.
   My friend also brought me a smiley balloon. Some days it
was the only smile in the house but it promised brighter days to
come.
   On the day I had exploratory surgery, another friend gave
me a goofy figurine. I was unexpectedly hospitalized afterwards

33

and that figurine reminded me of caring love all through the long night hours.

Ways to Bring a Smile

Never underestimate the power of a light-hearted moment. Medical research now shows the physical and emotional benefits of laughter. Sometimes we hold back from introducing humor in a situation out of concern that it will be inappropriate or taken poorly. And there are times that humor is not helpful.

So ask your friend for permission to have a lighthearted moment. Say:

"I heard a really awful groaner joke. Would you like to hear it?" Or:

"I was reading about the medical benefits of humor and I wonder if we could take a few moments from our regular time together to…" Or:

"I brought something really silly that I thought you might like to share with your family (or medical staff). May I show it to you?"

And if your friend isn't up to it, she'll say no and that's okay. In fact it empowers her. How many times in her medical treatment can she refuse something? But if she says yes, some things you might consider sharing are:

Silly Jokes

Take copies of printed silly jokes or cartoons to leave with her so she can share them with others. You can find them in books and online.

One knock knock joke that's good for her to share with medical staff is about HIPPA, those hospital rules that protect privacy by having people not share information. It goes:

Knock Knock. Who's there? HIPPA. HIPPA who? I can't tell you.

Chicken jokes are always popular:

Why did the chicken cross the basketball court? She heard the referee call a foul.

Why did the chicken cross the playground? To get to the other *slide.*

Why couldn't the chicken find her egg? She mislaid it.

At this point, you may be thinking that a silly joke doesn't do very much. But shifting her mind, even for a moment, is giving her a "breather" from the daily grind and reconnecting her to the lighter side of life.

Sometimes it can do even more. The late actor Christopher Reeve recalled how he laughed at fellow actor Robin Williams who visited him wearing a blue scrub hat, a yellow gown and speaking with a funny accent. Reeve is quoted as saying "I laughed for the first time (since my paralysis) and I knew that life was going to be okay."

Comedian Bob Hope has said "I have seen what a laugh can do. It can transform almost unbearable tears into something bearable, even hopeful."

Visual Props and Ideas

Find colorful, silly hats for you and your friend. On the internet, buy kazoos, rubber chickens and latex-free clown noses. Look for funny pictures of animals in magazines or in Youtube (www.youtube.com) videos.

Record or buy programs by her favorite comedians. Laughter has a long-shelf life. You can revisit a funny episode time and again and still enjoy the lighthearted lift. Norman Cousins, author of *Anatomy of an Illness* who watched Marx Brothers films said that "ten minutes of genuine belly laughter had an anesthetic effect and would give me at least two hours of pain-free sleep."

Look for humor in your own life to share. "A funny thing happened the other day…"

Celebrate milestones in her journey with fun mementos. Cut out paper "wings" and tape them to a crayon, telling her she passed her test (or ended her treatment) with "flying colors."

The Power of Mirth

In summary, know that your presence with your friend in times of sadness and joy will make a tremendous difference. Whenever possible, lighten her load with love and laughter.

Perhaps it is said best by this poem in Richard Snowberg's (out of print) book *The Caring Clowns: How Humor, Smiles and Laughter Overcome Pain, Suffering and Loneliness:*

> The value, the worth and the power of mirth
> Can help each of us to get through
> When the going is rough and incredibly tough,
> And even the sunshine looks blue,
> For once you give in to a chuckle or grin,
> Your spirits just natur'ly lift,
> And life is worthwhile each time that you smile,
> For a laugh is a God-given gift.

Anita Thies lives with her husband Jim, her dog Tasha and her flock of rubber chickens in State College, PA. She is co-author of **The Joyful Journey of Hospital Clowning: Making a Difference with Love and Laughter** *which may be downloaded for free at her website: www.tootheclown.com.*

The Lump and I –
What I've Learned From My Bout
With Breast Cancer
Anne Abayasekara

It may be that scores of women around Sri Lanka are fingering their breasts nervously at this moment to ascertain whether they can feel any unwelcome lumps.   I know three such, all of them about 30 years younger than I, who did discover lumps and were unutterably relieved to find they were benign or harmless. With the approach of my 85th birthday, I really thought I'd sailed past those perilous seas into calm waters, but I did continue to look for lumps. And then on Sunday, January 24th, I did discover one, although I half hoped it was my imagination. I kept mum about it until January 26th. when I asked a doctor friend of mine whether she would be good enough to have a look at my left breast and tell me whether the offending lump really existed. She kindly came over, examined me and said, "Yes, there definitely is a lump and you'd better have it out quickly, even though it's probably a harmless one, as I can't feel any glands."

The two questions that I am most frequently asked now are: "Does breast cancer occur in women over 80?" and, "How did you find out that you had a lump?" I've learned that breast cancer is by no means uncommon among us oldies – both my surgeon and an Oncologist confirmed this. The compensating factor is that among us old people, the cancer develops at a much slower rate than it does in the younger age group of 40s and 50s. "It's not so virulent," said my surgeon. As to how I discovered it, the habit of feeling my breasts for lumps at bath time was routine with me – not that anyone in my immediate family had suffered from breast or any other cancer, but because there's so much publicity given today to the need to look for lumps. However, my Oncologist emphasized that what every woman over 40 should do, is to have a Mammogram taken once a year, because by that means even a small "seed" is discovered long before it grows into an identifiable lump and if it is malignant or cancerous, early treatment is so much more effective. People make a big thing of a Mammogram being a painful procedure. May I state that while it does hurt when a lever is clamped down on your breast, the pain is of momentary duration, for just a minute or two, and is surely preferable to the suffering that can be caused by a full-blown cancer?

I saw a reputed surgeon on January 27. He examined me and murmured, "Yes, there is definitely a lump." He sent me for a Mammogram and a fine needle biopsy of the lump at a private hospital. The doctor who looked at my Mammogram ordered an Ultra-Sound scan as well. As for the fine-needle biopsy, I hardly felt the prick, although it had to be done a second time. The report was that I was clear and I felt pleased.

Since the fine needle biopsy cleared my lump of malignancy, my surgeon, Dr. G., recommended a lumpectomy the very next day. `Lumpectomy' means a fairly simple surgical procedure whereby the lump is removed under a local anesthetic. I went home in a couple of hours, having been given the "lump" (floating in a bottle of spirits) to be handed in for a biopsy.

We then informed my eldest daughter who happens to be an Oncologist practicing in New Jersey, USA. Ranmali was on the 'phone to me immediately. I told her the fine needle biopsy had cleared me, but she spoke candidly and was of the opinion that the lump was very likely to be malignant, as the fine needle procedure doesn't always give an accurate result. This deflated me somewhat. In the event, she was right and even before we got the biopsy report confirming Ranmali's suspicion, she arrived here in person and accompanied me on my next visit to Dr. G. He read the biopsy report and discussed what options I had. It was a huge relief to me and to all the family that Ranmali was present to guide us, in discussion with Dr. G. I was to have a full mastectomy of the left breast, with removal of lymph nodes. It all seemed unreal. I wasn't at all nervous, but felt as if it were happening to someone else.

I had my breast removed by Dr. G., under general anesthesia on February 8th, in the late evening – this is what is called a Mastectomy. Thirteen lymph nodes were also removed. When I regained consciousness I felt no pain whatsoever. It was nice the next morning, to have the ministrations of a most competent nursing attendant who gave me a wonderful sponge from head to toe. Nicer still, was the appetizing breakfast of stringhoppers with pol-sambol and a curry. I guessed I was on pain-killers and antibiotics when the nurses brought round pills of various shapes and hues and I am happy to declare that at no point did I have even a twinge of pain. I was able to get out of bed and go to the toilet on that first day.   I came home on the evening of Feb.11 and was able to come to the computer after dinner to send off an e-mail to Ranmali (who had gone back by then) and to my other children abroad, assuring them that I was doing fine.

While in hospital, I had a tube draining fluid from the wound into a bottle.   This was taken out the day before I left, but on two subsequent visits to Dr. G., he had to drain fluid again – this procedure, again, is hardly felt. I had stopped taking the pain-killers quite early on, with the surgeon's permission. On Feb. 21st, with the surgeon's blessing, I travelled to Kandy by car and on the 25th I was able to sit through SIX solid hours of the Peradeniya University's General Convocation 2009 at which my granddaughter was among the graduates.

Back in Colombo, I resumed my normal life. I've been to see the Oncologist, Dr. A., with whom Ranmali had spoken when she was here. He was as satisfied with my progress as my surgeon had been. He asked me whether I had started taking the pill, `Femara', which he knew Ranmali had brought me and he asked me to continue with that for a few years. No chemotherapy and no radiation. No dietary restrictions. I should see him every four months.

Ranmali gave us a very lucid account of my diagnosis and prognosis at a family conclave held round my dining table one day. I'd like to share with you some of what she said from a medical viewpoint, because it might be helpful. Although it is hoped that the removal of the breast lump would ensure a cure, sometimes the cancer "returns" because there are microscopic cells which have already escaped. These are not detectable and remain dormant, but can start growing at any point in time and show up as "metastases" in any part of the body. This could happen up to 30 years later in slow- growing situations, and much sooner in others. Four common factors are considered when assessing what the risk is and what can be done to prevent it. (1) Is there lymph-node involvement? (In my case, 2 out of 13 lymph nodes that were removed, had cancer cells – but the plus point is that these lymph nodes were taken out). (2) The size of the tumour. My lump was 2.5 cms. In general, if any tumour is more than 1 cm. some kind of treatment is recommended. (3) Was the tumour sensitive to Estrogen? This is measured by what is called the Estrogen Receptor and Progesterone Receptor. Mine were highly positive – 99% and 93% - and this is a GOOD thing for 2 reasons. The first is that in general, people with ER and PR positive tumours, have a better prognosis. The second is that because these tumours are sensitive to Estrogen (that is, Estrogen can make the tumour grow), by blocking the Estrogen, any microscopic cells that may be around can be "killed". This is the single most effective way one can prevent breast cancer from recurring. (4) A check is made for a protein called the HER2 protein. This was negative in my case, which was also a good sign as people with HER2 positive have a higher risk of recurrence.

I understand that since two of the lymph nodes that were removed were cancerous, cancer cells could be lurking undetected in some part of my body. In younger people, this would mean chemotherapy as well, but it has been found that in older people with ER positive tumours, the risk of recurrence is reduced by almost 50% with these Estrogen Blockers – I should take the tablet I am on, "Femara", for 5 years. In general, older people have slower-growing cancers. Ranmali explained to me that I don't need radiation since I had the mastectomy, but if my tumour (or lump) had been over 5 cms, or if more than 4 lymph nodes were positive (high risk), then Radiation would have been indicated. The down-side of the pill, Femara, is that it promotes Osteoporosis and X-rays have shown that I already suffer from this condition. In order to counteract this, I am also on a weekly pill called Osteofos 70, along with two tablets of calcium (Regucalcium) which I take daily.

Overall, my prognosis is fairly good, but, as Ranmali says, with cancer one never knows. One other point she stressed is that a positive outlook is always a plus point. I thank God that I am naturally a resilient type and I have plenty of interests to take my mind off disease. With cancer spreading around the world like global warming, I would add that having an Oncologist in the family is a big bonus!

"Courtesy of Sunday Times, Colombo"
Re-printed here with permission

Anne lives in Colombo, Sri Lanka. She has been a journalist her whole adult life. She is 86 years old and still contributes articles to newspapers as a free-lance journalist. Writing is what she most enjoys doing. She has one published book. ***"Hurrah! For Large Families"*** *which is about life with her brood of seven!*

Stitch by Stitch
Barbara Abbott

November 2010 was a life-changing experience when I found out I had inflammatory breast cancer. I began treatments in December after having surgery to install a port for the chemotherapy. It has been heart-warming to receive so many cards and prayers from even strangers who tell my husband and me that they are praying for my recovery every day! From the warm hugs I receive from a lady assistant store manager at the local grocery store to so many asking how I am doing and telling me to let them know if I need anything, I know I am not alone in this fight.

I have received two prayer shawls from a local group and a United Methodist church in Virginia. I know that each stitch was lovingly created with prayer for me. Two weeks ago, I received a beautiful red prayer quilt sent to me from a United Methodist Church in North Carolina. The quilt, when finished by a group of ten women in the church who make them, was placed on the altar during services. As church members prayed for me and my healing, they tied a knot in the quilt. When I look at that beautiful, hand-pieced quilt, I know that prayers went into each knot and each stitch, and I am thankful that God puts it on the hearts of His followers to extend kindness and caring to those who are so greatly in need.

I have known many family members and friends who have had cancer, some of whom survived and some of whom did not. Even that knowledge did not quite prepare me for the reality of what it means to actually be a person who is receiving chemotherapy. I knew it would be challenging, but nothing can quite prepare you for the nausea (which is better for current patients than it was years ago, thanks to drugs administered with the chemo), the weakness, fever, numbness of the fingers, pain in the feet, etc. Even walking down our driveway to the mail box is the limit of what I am able to do some days, when I often walked the 1/8 mile out to the family farm and back four or five times a day without even thinking about it.

I think one of the most distressing side effects for me has been the loss of taste; some of the foods and beverages I loved best now don't taste good to me. I was an avid Pepsi, Sierra Mist, and grape juice drinker -- now I find the cloying sweetness more than I can handle. I have become addicted instead to water with lemon juice and V-8 juice, because it lacks the sweetness of my former favorite drinks.

As a person who has always loved being around other people, another difficult thing for me has been the isolation of being too ill to go out, many days choosing to stay at home and watch TV or read on the living room couch with my two black Pugs, Roxie and Rambo. They know something is wrong with me, and their noses alert them when I've had chemo. Roxie was quite upset when I began losing my hair, and even after several months of seeing me bald, she still stares at me and lets me know she is worried at the change.

I moved one of my computers into the corner of the living room from my basement office, and began a new adventure of connecting with friends and family on Facebook. This was one of the best decisions I made for myself during this battle, as it allowed me to work on short stories for my publishing company without having to leave my "safe haven" in the living room. I can connect with the outside world at any hour day or night, which helps keep me from feeling as isolated as I might otherwise have done.

I decorated for the Christmas season early, realizing that I would not feel up to doing my usual sprucing up of the house after I began treatment. The themed Christmas trees in each room helped brighten the first few months, along with my collection of Christmas village houses displayed in several rooms. Finally, in early March, the long, cold winter urged me to slowly put them away, instead getting out silk flowers to turn my house into Spring.

This has been a good opportunity to stop and think about faith, about healing, about the God who cares so much for each of

His children. He is never far from me, and when I feel discouraged and alone, I know I am not, because God will never leave us. I have read many good Christian fiction books over the last few months, getting time to delve into the extensive library I have collected over the past several years. I have also shared some of those books with Amish friends and neighbors who are avid readers.

I am very thankful for the caring and compassion of the physicians, nurses and staff in the Geisinger Group at Scenery Drive. They are patient and kind, helping cancer patients through the most difficult time in their lives. After the first treatment, I was more comfortable, knowing what to expect during the chemotherapy as well as the side effects that follow during the first week or so. Answers to questions were only a phone call or email away.

Cancer is a humbling experience, a growing one, and one that lets you reach deep inside yourself for the real meaning of life and love of family and friends. One learns to not "sweat the small stuff," and that most of life really is "small stuff" when you compare it to the daily need to survive each moment, each hour, and each day. It teaches you the value of a cheery card, a caring phone call, the assurance of prayers for healing each and every day, even from strangers.

I know God wants the best for me as His child, and I am looking forward to a complete healing from the cancer. I believe God has a lot more for me to do, and I pray that I will use my remaining years wisely. Having gone through this experience, I am more aware of the pain and suffering in the world around me, the discouragement people feel, and the wonderful, uplifting help we can give to others by caring, praying, and sharing with them when they are going through a dark valley of illness, especially cancer.

Thank you, God, for being with me through this challenging time. Thank You for friends, family, my church family, and all those strangers who have been so kind and thoughtful. Thank you for another hour, another day, and another year to share Your love to others around me. Thank you for life, love, and happiness that comes from You even in the midst of the hardest times. We can make it -- because of Your love -- and knowing that our lives are really in Your hands, today and always. You turn our tears of discouragement, fear, pain and sorrow into joy, knowing that we are always in Your care.

Barbara lives in Madisonburg, PA, with her husband John and daughter Michelle. She is retired from Penn State, and writes regularly for Union Gospel Press of Cleveland, OH. You can reach her by email at: barbya1@yahoo.com.

A Sprinkle of FUN from Tammy...
Martha's Way or My Way...

Martha's Way: Don't throw out all that leftover wine. Freeze it into ice cubes for future use in casseroles and sauces.

My Way: What leftover wine?

Mamie
Erika Airhart

October 12, 2009 was a day that I will never forget. My grandmother, who I fondly called "Mamie," passed away after a long battle with breast cancer.

The time I spent with Mamie was definitely nowhere near what I would have liked, partly because up until 2007, we lived in other states while she lived in Pittsburgh. My father's job always seemed to relocate us at not-so-convenient times. However the latest move, in 2007 – "home" to Pittsburgh, would soon become the most important move of our lives.

In April of 2009, my husband and I discovered we were going to have a baby. It was the most exciting time of our lives and Mamie was one of the first people we told. Our due-date was late November. Mamie had already been diagnosed with breast cancer at this time and was undergoing treatment for it along with some other medical issues.

When she was first diagnosed with breast cancer she made the decision not to undergo chemotherapy or have any surgeries. Instead, her doctor prescribed her Tykerb which she would take daily. Mamie never had a driver's license or learned to drive so my mom took her prescription to the pharmacy to be filled. When she went to pick it up she was told the cost for a one-month supply would be $3,000. There was no way this would be a viable option every month. Her doctor contacted the pharmaceutical company and they agreed to help out and cover most of the medication cost for her. She would thankfully only need to pay $35 each month for this live-sustaining drug.

From 2006 through 2009, she had a few hospital stays for various medical reasons – but then in the summer of 2009 she started having more severe health problems, which were complicated further by the breast cancer. There were days when I would be afraid to answer my phone once I saw my mom's name on the caller-ID. I dreaded hearing her say Mamie was in the hospital or that they had to call the ambulance for her.

Mamie was so worried about me going to visit her during any of the times she was in the hospital. She was more concerned with my pregnancy and the risks associated with being around sick people in the hospital. It was a very frustrating time. I relied heavily on daily updates from my mom as to how she was doing and how her treatments were going. My pregnancy was going great but unfortunately Mamie's health was doing the exact opposite.

By August she had been back and forth so many times between her home and the hospital that the decision was made for her to go to a live-in facility. By this time she was having difficulty speaking but she made it through each day. My mom spent every day with her, from when she was in the hospital to the live-in facility. My mom is the reason Mamie made it through each day. She didn't have time to worry about herself – she spent her days worried about me, her only child who was going to have a baby, and her own Mother.

Mamie's health took a turn for the worst in September. The few times she was able to speak, she would ask to "go home". She had always been rather skinny and looked frail, but now she looked like she could break if anyone spoke too loudly and their breath reached her. In her last days, her nurses told my mom that it would be safe for me to come visit her and spend some time with her.

The first visit to see her in the live-in facility felt like a dream. I tried to prepare myself with what to expect and remind myself to ignore the machines that would be in her room. As soon as I got in the room, all I could think about was Mamie. I wanted to take her pain away and make her healthy again. I was mad at the cancer for taking so much from Mamie and our whole family.

Once Mamie's health started declining, it deteriorated quickly and my mom began difficult discussions with the doctors about what we should do. Mamie did not want to have machines keeping her alive, which was the way things were at this point. The decision was made to turn off the machines and let her finally "go home".

October 12, 2009, my family and I gathered in her small hospital room; my mom, my dad, my husband, 3 of my aunts, and one of my uncles. The nurse came in and turned off Mamie's ventilator. My heart hoped that she would start breathing on her own. My mind prayed that this was all a dream and that I would wake up in my comfy bed. I stood next to Mamie's bedside, fighting back tears and holding her hand, as she took her last breaths. The days that followed were surreal but despite the pain we felt in our hearts, we had a baby to still prepare for.

On November 19th, 2009 Christopher Michael was born into this world. He was a feisty little baby from the start; just like his Great-Mamie. We knew from the moment he was born that Mamie passed away before he was born for a reason. Christopher was born with little birthmark on his left ear, as if Mamie had kissed him good-bye before sending him to us. She may have passed away but she is with us every day; in memory, in spirit, in Christopher.

Erika lives in Crafton, PA with her husband, Adam, and their almost 2-year-old son, Christopher. She works full-time in finance and loves spending time with her family, crafting, sewing, watching/playing sports and volunteering. You can reach her at: erika.airhart2011@gmail.com

A Sprinkle of FUN from Tammy…
Martha's Way or My Way…

Martha's Way: When a cake recipe calls for flouring the baking pan, use a bit of the dry cake mix instead and there won't be any white mess on the outside of the cake.

My Way: Go to the bakery. They'll even decorate it for you.

Christine Allen

Imagine
Christine Allen

There I was, standing in front of a whole group of women, their faces smiling at me and there was pink everywhere. I was telling my story at the State conference of the PA Breast Cancer Coalition. That is something I could have never imagined...

Imagine holding a "secret" inside of you for over 31 years. Imagine that "secret" is something that almost everyone talks about these days, but you were forbidden to even breathe the words. For me, that "secret" was that I was diagnosed with breast cancer.

It was a very different time in 1975. I worked for the local school district as a cook from 1965 until 1993. When I was diagnosed in 1975 with breast cancer, I did not dare breathe a word to anyone that I had breast cancer. At that time, many people thought it was highly contagious and was even compared to people with AIDS. People thought that you could "spread" cancer by touching someone. If I had told anyone, it would have certainly meant the end to my job, and as a single mother of three beautiful children, I could not risk being unemployed. In fact, the word cancer was rarely spoken, but it was referred to as the "Big C".

Fortunately, if you can say that, I had problems with my back, so when I had to be off for cancer surgery and recovery, I just told people it was because of my back problems. I didn't really get sick, my recovery was fairly good, and that was a good thing. My doctor was the only one who knew what was really happening.

I found the lump while I was doing an exam in the shower. It was a tiny, tiny little thing, about the size of a pin head. When I had it checked, they tried to aspirate it but they couldn't get anything. The doctor tried again, and when he gave me the results, he didn't even sit down. He came into the room and just said, Christine, it is cancer", and he walked out of the room! I was in a complete daze and didn't know which way to turn or what to do.

49

As fate would have it, I had JUST read a story about a doctor, Dr. Carl Mansfield, who was the first black man to head up the Radiology Dept. at Thomas Jefferson Hospital. I didn't know what I was thinking, but I walked right over to that hospital to the Radiology department and asked if I could see him! The nurse went to get him and he came out to see me! Imagine that! Dr. Mansfield said he wasn't able to help me, but he would get a doctor who could help. That doctor turned me over to another doctor, a female doctor, and I was finally with a doctor who cared about me as a patient – the whole me, not just the cancer.

Although I didn't say a word to anyone, I started talking to a lot of women that I knew who had breast cancer. ALL, yes every one of them told me that they lost their breast, or both breasts during their surgery, and they didn't know until they woke up in the recovery room. My doctor was a female and just out of medical school a couple of years. When I mentioned this to her, she said that she didn't do it this way. She believed at the time that a lot of doctors just didn't care about the after affects of a breast removal – they just did it. The word I remember her using was "radical". She said there was a new procedure that she used and IF they had to take my breast, she would wake me up before she did it. As it turned out, the cancer was small, stage 1, and I was able to keep my breast.

I was off work for just a couple of weeks. After the surgery, I went to the library and read everything I could find about chemotherapy and radiation. At that time there was very little that a person could find that was in language that a regular person could understand. Certainly nothing like what is available to people today.

I attended every seminar I could find where they were talking about cancer and it seemed like the idea of your health and your diet came out in a lot of them. My doctor told me once that we are all born with cells that could lead to cancer, it was just the choice of cells which way they went and whether they became cancer.

I was always interested in alternative medicines so I went to a little store on Green Street in Philadelphia, PA, called Penn Herbs and met with Lonzo. Penn Herbs is still there in Philadelphia!! He talked to me at great length and made up a variety of herbs, drops, teas, and pills for me to take. He told me to go to the doctor and listen to everything they told me, then tell him and he would duplicate what I needed.

You can believe what you like, but for me, I know without a doubt that I was healed because I believe in two things – prayer and Jesus!

During the recovery time, I think I felt "lost" because I couldn't talk to anyone about anything that was going on. I certainly had the Lord, or maybe I should say He had me. The whole process was a very frightening experience because I didn't have anyone to help me through or really be able to discuss it with anyone except my doctor. Someone asked me once if I felt I had any special treatment with my cancer. I told them "no" because no one knew anything about it! I was always on guard for fear that someone would find out. I had a neighbor across the street who helped me from time to time with groceries, but she had done that before the cancer so it was no different.

I would love to say that was the end of breast cancer in my life, but the Lord had other plans. In 2004, my beautiful daughter Pauline, at age 52, came home and told me she was diagnosed with breast cancer. As she was filling out the papers for her treatment, she made a statement that it was interesting that there was no family history. It was as if the dam broke and I told her, *for the very first time*, that I had breast cancer 31 years before!

I have been asked many times why I never said anything before that time to anyone. I can't honestly say whether it was shame or it was just forgotten or maybe I still had a little fear of what might happen. I still didn't tell her all the details of what I went through, but just that I had cancer. Again, I don't know why but I think it was hidden so deep inside all of those years, I just couldn't. Whatever the reason, Pauline and my family were hearing it for the first time.

Pauline's cancer was found during a mammogram. She knew very early that it was cancer and was given a lot of information regarding her options. What a difference from my diagnosis! I vividly remember feeling like I was numb and in a daze and asked Pauline if she was okay. She said she was fine and felt like she was very informed.

Pauline's story has a different outcome than mine. She did the chemo and radiation. During one of the visits to have her port changed, something happened, which to this day NO ONE has been able to figure out, but Pauline contracted some type of bacteria. She was in the hospital for three days, and then went into a coma for six weeks. It settled in her back and she is now confined to a wheelchair. Everyone, I mean everyone tried to check everything and there just isn't any explanation for what happened, but I am thankful I still have my daughter and I was glad I was there to help care for her while she was in the hospital. I knew what she needed and I was able to be there for her, to be her voice.

Through all the challenges, God has blessed us abundantly! I have three wonderful children, five grandchildren and six great-grandchildren and life is very full! Many members of my family have been educated and serve in positions where they help other people. I am very proud of all of them!

Tammy asked me to talk about what I had learned through all of this and what I tell people today. I have a few things I would like to share with you that may or may not be helpful.

First, we need to PRAY and talk to God the same way we talk to our very best friend. He knows all about us, no matter what. Sometimes we need to wait and sometimes the answer is no, but we must always pray and talk to Him.

Second, do not ever give up! There is always hope and we must never give up hope! I am a 36 year survivor and I never gave up hope.

Third, you have to trust your gut. Your gut can help you in a lot of ways, not just trusting. Our diet and health, what we put in our gut is very important. We need to eat healthy to keep our system regular and keep our gut clean and working. I firmly believe in green tea and yogurt as two ways to keep us healthy. We need to eat more grains and fiber, especially whole grains and the darker the breads the healthier. Put good things in your body. I believe that if I had eaten better throughout my life I would not be dealing with high blood pressure and diabetes, and who knows, maybe I wouldn't be writing this story as a breast cancer survivor.

Fourth, we MUST take a hand in our own health, not just being informed while we are making decisions and going through things, but also afterwards to make sure we are doing everything we can to maintain our health. We have to get second opinions, and learn everything we can about our options. If you don't like your doctor, especially, if she/he doesn't treat you as a whole person, not just the ailment or disease, then get another doctor – your doctor has to be good for you! For example, with cancer chemo may be an option, but it may not be the only option. Be vigilant. Do regular breast exams. Get plenty of rest.

Fifth, along with your doctor you have to choose a hospital that has love and YOU in mind! You can't treat cancer separate from the whole person. They have to love you and be there for you!

If you need help, then ASK for it. I couldn't go to any support groups because I was so afraid that someone would find out. Pauline went to support groups and they even asked her to bring her family along because they were part of the recovery. I never had anything like that. There are a lot of people out there to help – ask for it and seek out what YOU need.

Not too long ago I had another scare. The doctors thought they found something again and I went through more tests. There was definitely something that they both found, but when they went back, they couldn't find anything on the films. I told them they can call it whatever they like, but I call it Jesus! When Jesus heals you, it's a promise. What He does, lasts, and there is power in His healing!

Imagine! For so many, many years I was unable to open my mouth about my life and what was going on, and now, with

Him glory and blessing, I am using my voice to try and help others! Amazing grace, indeed!

Christine Allen
As written by Tammy Miller

Christine Allen lives in Philadelphia and is a 73 year young mother of three; grandmother of five; and great-grandmother of six beautiful children. She works with the Wellness Community, which just merged with the Gilda Radner Foundation, to help other people facing the challenges of cancer. She was awarded the "Champion of Inspiration" award from the Susan G. Komen Foundation, and is deeply involved in volunteering efforts, most recently with the hospice program at the University of Pennsylvania. She works with the Community Health Center #5 of the Philadelphia Department of Health and serves as a Board member and volunteer. Author's note: And, she was an inspiration for this book!

Changing Times (Thankfully)
Cynthia Anderson

In 1981, I went after work one day for my first mammogram. It was a terrible experience. The office was cold, dreary and unwelcoming and the people were unfriendly. I put the vest that they give you on backwards, was then ridiculed by the technician and just felt that the entire visit was humiliating. When I left that day, I swore that I would never go back for another mammogram again – and I didn't, for sixteen years.

After a decade and a half, I received a letter from my insurance company "reminding" me that I hadn't gone for a mammogram in years. Truthfully, my initial thought was that the letter was rude and it was none of their business. I kept the letter, though, and after a while began to worry that maybe they would cancel my insurance because of it. So, completely unenthusiastic, I scheduled an appointment for a mammogram.

I was shocked at how much everything had changed since my first visit. The people were accommodating and friendly, and the office was warmer with colored wallpaper and decorations. The whole experience was so much better, until the bad news started.

I was told they found micro-calcifications on my mammogram that are indicators of early breast cancer and from there, everything happened very quickly. I had an excisional biopsy, which confirmed the diagnosis followed by immediate surgery, and went back to work right away. I opted not to have reconstruction. At that time, it was very hard to find prostheses and I was extremely frustrated. Eventually I found a small shop that sold them. Years later, larger clothing stores ultimately began offering these types of things as well.

Since my experience, people have become much more open when speaking about the disease. I remember, before I was diagnosed, I met a woman who was surprisingly forthcoming about her breast cancer. I used to make the daily deposits for the municipality and she was the person who processed them; that was the extent of our relationship. I always thought it was so strange when she would talk to me about her cancer and mastectomy. All I could really think was, "we're in a bank, for goodness sake." As time went on, though, I came to truly admire her and how she dealt with her disease. After being diagnosed myself, it solidified my opinion that talking openly about your cancer is a good thing. A woman who lived down the street from me was also diagnosed and had completely secluded herself for months; she did not want to talk to anyone about what she had gone through. One day, I thought "the heck with it" and knocked on her door to ask her to talk. We spoke for a while about her cancer and mastectomy; she cried for the first time that day, and finally came to terms with her situation. Today, she is a gracious, confident woman.

Having my daughter diagnosed last year was a completely different story. I was devastated for her and struggled to process her diagnosis. Although she had regular checkups for years, her cancer was much more advanced. She needed chemotherapy and eventually radiation. I wanted to ease her "chemo days" and the fatigue it created, so I made weekly visits with prepared meals and helped with laundry and other tasks around the house. Watching her struggle with the indignities she was forced to endure as a result of her chemotherapy broke my heart. Her sense of humor, strength of character, and wonderful support from her husband and family got her through the trying times. Today, I am so very proud of her and the tremendous strides she's made. She is a beautiful lady.

Cynthia Anderson
As written by Kelsey Itak (her granddaughter and a Pink Ribbon Writer for this book)

Cynthia Anderson lives in Point Pleasant Beach, NJ with her husband. She has 4 children, 8 grandchildren, and 3 step-grandchildren.

Attitude Is Everything
Pam Asencio

It was mid afternoon on Wednesday, November 4th 2009, and I had just written a $615 check for breast cancer research. I raised this money from two fundraisers I did using my home-based business. I put the check in the mailbox and went to shower as my one-year old daughter napped. As I'm showering I find a lump and instantly my mind was racing. Could it, no it couldn't…I just had a mammogram in July and it was clear.

Hourly I would check to see if it was still there and it was. How had I not felt this before? I'm sure it is nothing. My husband makes me promise that if I still feel it in the morning, I need to call my doctor immediately. Well, I called for an appointment that day and saw my doctor that day. She felt it and immediately thought it was a cyst. To be safe, she immediately got me scheduled for a mammogram which showed no lump. This was very strange because we could easily feel it. So, my doctor scheduled an ultrasound. The ultrasound confirms the lump and that it is not a cyst. The radiologist thinks fibro adenoma, but decides that we should do a biopsy to be sure. The biopsy is scheduled for a week later on Friday the 13th.

Now it is the waiting game. I was supposed to be celebrating my 40th birthday in 3 days with friends – football and fun – but now I'm just going through the motions pretending to smile while a dark cloud looms over my head. My husband, Dave, and I decided to only tell a few people as we do not want our children to worry until we know the facts. The biopsy came and went and now more waiting…I truly believe waiting is the most difficult part of your journey as you try to stay positive and fail miserably at it. My way to beat the waiting game was to schedule myself beyond busy with life, work, and family.

I vividly remember C-Day…the day I received the call that I had cancer – breast cancer. The doctor and I had been playing phone tag and my anxiety and stress were at an all time high. My husband, Dave came home knowing I would be receiving the return call soon. It came and the doctor told me I had breast cancer and then the next question she asks catches me off guard. My doctor asks if I'm surprised by this information that it is breast cancer. Of course I'm surprised. I just turned 40, I exercise daily, I take care of myself, I get my yearly exams and mammograms and I am feeling great! This one call changed my life forever.

I hung up the phone and began to crumble. I turned to Dave who was also crying and I instantly began to think of not living to see my kids grow up. Dave looked straight into my eyes and said I had one day to feel sorry for myself and then it was time to put my game face on, become a warrior and fight the most important battle in my life. He said to me "promise me just one thing – that you will fight this 110% every single minute of every day. If you do that, you win. And you will win!"

Let the fight begin…this was a battle for me, my husband, my three children (Sydney age 9, Matthew age 6 and Samantha age 1 at the time of diagnosis), my parents and for everyone who had touched my life. I would not let them down. We were going to beat this and this is where attitude comes into play. Attitude is EVERYTHING! We chose to BELIEVE, to fight, and to win. Losing was not an option. Each day, I chose to take the positive road and I would not allow the cancer to consume or control me. For my family and for myself I wanted to keep our schedule as normal as possible. During chemotherapy and multiple surgeries, I would continue to work, exercise and attend all my kid's activities.

I had the genetic testing done during chemo to find out if I had the breast cancer gene. We thought this call would come in weeks, came in days. I have the gene…BRCA2 gene. 80% chance of reoccurrence and over 40% chance of getting ovarian cancer. Now we have new data and it is time for a new plan of action. The new plan…once I have recovered from chemo, I would then have a bilateral mastectomy, reconstruction and the removal of my ovaries and tubes (ophorectomy). This decision was the best and only way I knew how to fight and WIN. We kept moving forward by referring to each appointment, surgery, treatment, follow-up, etc. as a box to check on our checklist.

When something was done, we checked it off our list and we were that much closer to the end.

I have been declared cancer free! I used to sweat the small stuff, but not so much anymore. I try to live in the present. I try to remain positive with everything in life. And, I fully intend to continue to pay it forward. Paying it forward is huge for me. I would have never gotten through this year long fight without the tremendous outpouring of support I received from family, friends, colleagues and even perfect strangers! I received encouraging emails and cards, thoughtful care packages, pajama grams, meals, help with my children and so much more. We all fought this battle together and WON!

A little Q & A with Pam…

Question:
What lessons have you learned along this journey?
Answer:
Don't sweat the small stuff. Be present. Attitude is everything. Trust your instincts. Pay it forward.

Question:
Was there anything along the path that surprised you?
Answer:
The biggest surprise to me was the complexity associated with diagnosing which type of breast cancer you have. Even though my mom is a two time breast cancer survivor, I had no idea about invasive, non-invasive, hormone receptive, triple negative, grades, etc. All of these things along with tumor size determine staging and treatment. When you take all of these complex factors into account, there is a myriad of options available for treatment. Also, since my mom never had chemotherapy, it never occurred to me that I might need it. Unfortunately, I was wrong.

Question:
Anything you wish your doctor would've told you?
Answer:
We now have a pill that you can take that will cure you.

Question:
What words of encouragement do you have to offer others?
Answer:
Believe. There is always something or someone worse off than you…you are blessed.

Pam Ascencio
As written By Kathy Salloum

Pam Asencio lives in Port Matilda, PA with her husband and 3 children ages 11, 8 and 3. She is an independent representative for Silpada Designs Jewelry and can be reached at pamasencio@comcast.net. BELIEVE!!!

Dancing Shoes
Gloria Benninghoff

When a woman hears the words "breast cancer", there are a lot of things that go through her mind. How will I tell my family? What will happen next? What type of recovery will I face? And, there is a lot of preparation to go to the hospital - gown, robe, toothbrush, and of course, my dancing shoes! And so my journey began…

It was the mid 1970's, I was just 38 years old, and I felt a lump in my breast while I was showering. After several mammograms, the lump was removed and determined to be an 8 cm benign cyst that was discovered just before it was ready to burst. This lump was benign but another lump was discovered in the same breast that was not felt before. This lump turned out to be cancer. I can never be sure, but I have always wondered if the radiation from the mammograms "fertilized" the lump.

Regardless of what created it, I now had to deal with all of the challenges of having breast cancer. At the time I had five children to take care of, with my youngest being very small, and my oldest daughter had just finished nursing school. I immediately sat the children down and explained what was happening as best as I could. I was concerned that if I didn't tell them, someone else would and may even tell them something that I didn't want them to hear, so I decided it was best for them to hear it from me.

Looking back over all of those years I don't think I ever thought I wouldn't make it through. With all of the children, I don't think the thought crossed my mind, there was simply too much that needed to be done. No matter what, I knew I was going to give it the best fight possible, because my children were depending on me. (A funny side story is that as I was preparing for this project, I found out my daughter wasn't going to entertain any other option either because she didn't want to get stuck raising the other children – she just told me that after all of this time!)

At the time of my surgery, there was a new two-step process that was being explored and it was very new to my community. The idea was that a woman could be given a choice as to what type of surgery she would want, dependent on the type and extent of the cancer. Before this time, a woman would go into surgery and have no idea whether or not she would have breasts when she awoke from surgery. This new process gave her a choice after the initial surgical diagnosis. It is common practice now, thankfully, but at that time it was still a new concept. I had to hold my ground that this was what I wanted and I became the first woman in my community to have this important, empowering decision for women.

There was a very calming event that happened during my surgery. What you choose to believe is up to you, but I can assure you this is exactly what happened, and I can recall it just as clearly today, all these years later, as if it had just happened. As I was taken into the operating room, I had a wonderful sense of peace. I clearly, without ANY question, saw Jesus behind me. When my doctor came in he told me that "I was very special" as he never operated alone, but this particular day he would be. I just smiled at him and told him not to worry, that he wasn't operating alone this day either!

Now, back to the dancing shoes! When I checked into the hospital I did have the gown, robe and toothbrush, and the dancing shoes! My theory was that I was going to get through the surgery just fine and I would be out dancing again very soon. I used the dancing shoes as a visualization that the surgery was a necessity, but that I was going through it and out the other side with great success. I was in the hospital for 10 days, which is unheard of today, but each day I looked at those shoes as a literal "step" closer to recovery. During the days and weeks after the surgery I would sit on the bed and try on those dancing shoes. It took a little while, but one day the shoes went on and I went dancing!

I live in a small community and it doesn't take long for people to find out what may be happening with their neighbors. My experience was no different. It was interesting to recall that there was a stigma associated with cancer that people would shy away from you when they heard the word cancer. There was less understanding of the disease at the time and many people thought it was contagious. I believe others just do not know what to say to someone dealing with cancer so they don't say anything.

I have always found symbolism in many things in the world around me. Through the years butterflies have offered a symbol of hope. After the surgery I had a butterfly land directly on me. It was another reminder that what was happening was bigger than me and it offered peace and hope that all was happening for a reason and it would be fine.

After my surgery, my doctor put me on Alkeran. At that time, there wasn't as much information available to women and we tended to question less and just do whatever our doctor told us to do. Regardless, I just knew that this medication was going to take care of everything and I visualized strong, healthy healing and recovery. I was on the medication for one year when my doctor took me off Alkeran amidst the reports that it never really worked anyway. I don't know if it was the medication, visualization, or a strong faith, but this was just part of my healing process.

There were challenging days in the healing process, of course, but throughout it all we looked for reasons to laugh. In the same way that the power of the mind works, I am a firm believer in the power of laughter. We are always looking for a reason to laugh and have a great time, and I believe strongly that it can make any situation better. There is great value in understanding what we can change and what is out of our control. Knowing the difference between the two, and using humor and laughter in every situation can make a huge difference on healing and those around us.

I have learned a great deal about life since that first diagnosis. After all these years, it may be hard to believe but I still think some people are afraid and shy away from someone with cancer. I don't think as many believe it is contagious as they once did, but there still seems to be some of that. For whatever reason, it is a shame as this is a time when people need understanding, love and a warm touch so very much. This experience has had a great impact on my life and when I hear of someone dealing with cancer, I try to reach out and let them know they are not alone, and that there are many who care. We must ASK how we can help someone. Sometimes they don't even know yet, but please ask, reach out and be there for each other.

All things that happen in our lives are for a purpose. Sometimes we understand that purpose and sometimes we just don't. I keep saying that I am still trying to find my purpose in life. When I say that, my son always gives me a sly grin and says at my age I had better find my purpose pretty soon! When something like breast cancer happens to us we have a choice to become bitter or better, and it is our choice.

We are all in this life together and we must be there for each other to offer love, understanding and strength. Maybe we can send a card, or a thoughtful gesture, a phone call or a loving touch. Maybe someone just needs to know we care. Whatever we can do to help one another is vital. Or maybe, it is just to put on our dancing shoes and take someone dancing!

This story is dedicated to our forever angel, Ryleigh.

Gloria Benninghoff
As written by Tammy Miller

Gloria lives in State College, PA. She is a young 79 and has four wonderful children, a girl Jancie and 3 boys Richard, Kerry, Todd. She has been blessed with many loving friends and her precious Golden Retrievers.

MY CANCER STORY
(Sarah) Joanne Berkley

It started out with a nagging pain in my lower left side. When it went on for several weeks, I began to think about a doctor visit. I had had a hysterectomy back in 1980 but because of my age they had not removed my left ovary. With all the talk about ovarian cancer, I decided I had better have it checked out. On September 17, 2009 I had a female exam and pap smear. The doctor ordered a sonogram of my ovary which was done on Sept. 23, 2009. She also ordered blood work and, at the time, she asked if I wanted to have a mammogram since I hadn't had one for 2 years. I told her,"Okay, we might as well do it all" and she scheduled it .

The technician who did the mammogram on Oct. 3, 2009 was very thorough….I thought a little too thorough as I was not a big fan of mammograms, but I left happy to have it over with. Later that week I received a call that my x-ray was abnormal and they wanted to re-do it. I was assured by many of my friends that this had happened to them also and everything was fine. So I went back on Oct. 14, 2009 ready to hear that all was well. Not so….the person who read the x-rays was present and when they were all finished, I was told I needed to see a cancer surgeon. Strangely enough, I was calm and had no fear whatsoever. I thought, "How strange. I should be falling apart."

On Oct. 28, 2009 I had a consultation visit with Dr. Garguilo. He showed me on the x-rays, the spot they suspected was cancer and said a biopsy would need to be done to be sure. I had the biopsy at Johnstown Memorial Hospital on Nov. 18, 2009. The test results came back—cancer! Still...no fear. I had the peaceful feeling that everything was going to be okay.

On Dec. 9, 2009 I met with Dr. G. to discuss my options. Because of the small size of the lump, he said that a lumpectomy would be the best way to surgically remove it, and we scheduled my surgery for January 4, 2010. He also told me that I would be a candidate for a new way of doing radiation treatments but it was only done at the Indiana hospital. He would put a balloon in my breast after he removed the lump to hold a space for the catheter needed for the radiation treatments which would be twice a day for 5 days and I would be done. Wonderful! I checked with my insurance and everything was good to go.

In the meantime I had to have several scans to be sure there were no other cancers in my body plus blood work and consultation with the anesthesiologist.

On Monday, January 4, 2010, Dr. G. removed the lump from my breast along with several lymph nodes under my right arm. Testing on the nodes showed no spread of cancer cells there so I would only need to have radiation treatments—not chemo, so my stay at Indiana, PA was on.

I returned home the afternoon of January 4th with only a band-aid on my wound. My daughter (who drove me to the hospital) and I stopped at Wal-mart for a quick shopping trip on the way home.

On Wednesday January 6th, 2010, I drove myself to Lee Campus of Conemaugh Memorial Hospital for Dr. G. to remove the balloon and insert the catheter. I then drove myself to Indiana Regional where I was supposed to begin radiation treatments. Upon arrival, I found there was a slight problem….the machine needed was being serviced and wouldn't be ready until the following week.

I was very disappointed because the roads were icy and snow covered (being wintertime) but I decided to journey back home. Early Monday morning, January 11, 2010, I began receiving radiation treatments as planned. Dr. Tunio and the staff at the Cancer Center were wonderful. I returned home on Friday.

Since that time I have continued to have follow-up visits with Dr. Tunio and Dr. G. I've had mammograms (still not one of my favorite tests but one I highly recommend!) which have all been normal.

I have been cancer free now for over a year. Although I don't know why I had to have cancer, my faith is in God who made me, who has ordered all my days, and in his Son, Jesus

Christ, who died on the cross so that I might live with Him eternally.   He gave me peace, and led me to the right people to help me. This life is not all there is, so whether I am cured or die of cancer and go home to heaven, I WIN!

Joanne lives in Meyersdale, PA where she is part-time Secretary of the Grace Brethren Church, Treasurer of the Meyersdale Area Union Cemetery, and holds down a fulltime job at First National Bank. She is a widow with 5 grown children, eleven grandchildren, and one great, grandson. You may reach her at sjberkley@verizon.net

A Sprinkle of FUN from Tammy…

"I have everything I had twenty years ago, only it's all a little bit lower."   -- Gypsy Rose Lee

Sallie's Story
Sallie Boggs

My experience with breast cancer taught me the value of friends, the importance of taking action to get immediate and excellent care, to keep a sense of humor during treatment and then forget it.

I found my own little lump about the size of a bean. It was so small that my regular doctor could not feel it and she reluctantly ordered a mammogram. Neither did the mammogram show anything. Luckily, the mammogram technician could feel what I felt and ordered a sonogram. There it was, as clear as could be!

The results of the biopsy that followed were reported to my doctor and it was two weeks before she called me about it. By then I was already moving toward treatment. This was thanks to the technician who had agreed to call me as soon as the biopsy results came in. She actually confused me a bit by reporting that the biopsy was positive. When I said, "good" she said, "No, bad. Positive means that it is invasive cancer and you should see about treating it immediately."

Now you might think I could take this very rationally because I was a cancer researcher at the University of Pittsburgh School of Medicine, however, all I could think of was those invasive cancer cells doubling in my breast and I wanted them gone, now. I called a friend and collaborator who is an active breast cancer treatment doctor and he said I needed three specialists, a surgeon, a chemo therapist and a radiotherapist and he offered to make the appointments. I was sooo relieved. After appointments with all of them, the consensus was that for my stage-one lump a lumpectomy with radiotherapy and the new drug, Arimidex, total cure was very likely.

The doctors were all very careful to do all the important tests and explain things to me. I asked many questions and on advice of a book by my friend Tammy, I recorded all our conversations and listened to them when, inevitably, I forgot some detail. I had called Tammy immediately after I got my diagnosis to get her book and she sent both the book and a bag of red clown noses.

These noses got me through the surgery. I, my friend, and the hospital escort who pushed me from station to station in a wheel chair, all wore clown noses. There were two kinds of people we passed or interacted with. One group looked away as if they were embarrassed for us. The other group smiled or laughed out loud and waved or gave a thumbs-up. This little bit of levity lowered my anxiety and made it easier for my companions as well.

After the surgery, I was wheeled out to the waiting room to check out. I put on my clown nose and I turned to the many waiting breast cancer patients and, pointing to the nose I said, "I came in to have this removed and they took out a chunk of breast instead." Sure enough about half to them laughed.

I am 6 years out now from that day and am still taking Arimidex and still having the resultant hourly hot flashes. The other unpleasant side effects are gone. I had a scare last year when an artifact in the other breast was seen on a mammogram, but biopsy proved it to be benign. These days, I rarely think about breasts or cancer.

Thanks to friends and ever improving treatment and diagnostic techniques breast cancer can be little more than a temporary blip in your life. Be diligent in checking for lumps. If you find one, get it checked. If it is positive, find the best therapists, who work together and treat breast cancer every day, hold on to your friends and your sense of humor and it does not have to be a tragedy at all.

Sallie lives in a cottage with a view of the ocean at Birch Bay Retirement Village, Bar Harbor, ME. She shares the cottage with her long time partner Edward Redgate and standard poodle, Shanti. Her hobby is playing the stock market and walking in Acadia National Park with Ed, his 91 year old brother Ted and the dog. She recently started a Toastmasters club so she did not have to drive an hour to get to one.

Light After the Storm
Scott Boyd

May 10th 1974…It rained. A cold drenching rain fell.
Heaven wept as friends and family gathered to say goodbye to an
angel. The weather was fitting. So alone, at fifteen years old I
watched a casket descend into the cold dark earth. I hurt so bad, I
hugged myself. She was gone.

As people milled about our home offering words of
sympathy after the funeral everything seemed a haze. Late in the
afternoon, a friend asked if I'd walk with her to her car. She
wasn't obvious about it, but I know she prayed. Many prayed for
me. As I stood thanking her for the love and concern, the cold
gray sky broke…distant in the west the setting sun penetrated the
dark clouds beaming light and shadows. Between the horizon and
a sky dark and gray was a sliver of hope. Light after the storm…

"Honey, your mom has breast cancer." Six words that
smashed into the life of a 13-year-old boy! At 40 years old, June
Marie Haverstick Boyd looked at her youngest son and said, "don't
worry…everything will be ok." But the shake in her voice spoke
more fear than confidence.

The year was 1972. I was in 8th grade. Nixon was
president. The Viet Nam war was over. All was well in the
Universe, and I was in the center. Till now. I had never heard of
breast cancer. I didn't know what it was. I would soon learn.

I probably lived as close to a perfect life as any child could
enjoy. My parents were fantastic. I had a mom who loved
unconditionally, a dad who gave continuously. We enjoyed
summers at the pool, vacations at the beach, a great house,
fantastic friends and wonderful neighbors. Seriously…life was
GREAT.

Then, those 6 words. Nothing could prepare for what
would follow. Surgery, a radical mastectomy. Something thirteen
year olds don't really need to understand. But I had to. Radiation,
chemo-therapy—very experimental treatment at the time. Hair
loss, nausea and vomiting. Not just a 24 hour bug, but weeks. My

brother was off to college, my dad was back to work, and I was home watching as nurses and neighbors worked to bring healing.

Eventually the treatments seemed to work. The wigs and gowns were replaced with fresh new hair, and new clothes. In fact, mom actually went back to work.

Healing…Maybe?

And then the real cruelty began. A second lump in the remaining breast. Another mastectomy, more chemo, and radiation. Drugs and suffering. Candidly it was all a blur. There were more surgeries, and treatments and pain and suffering…and then somewhere in 1974, it became apparent that hope was fading. The only prayer was a miracle.

May 6, 1974 June Marie Boyd rested. She was freed from years of suffering. For her, Peace. But for a survivor, life became a storm. I existed in a sea of gray. I grew up fast, and I grew up hard. June of '74 through June of '77 was TOUGH. The loneliness is hard to describe, the pain at times unbearable. Words are simply not adequate.

But miracles happen.

They are mysterious and sometimes they are difficult to see. And seldom do they come as we expect, desire or demand. And just like that moment when the sky breaks at sunset, just after the storm, so miracles often appear in that sliver of space and time, between the horizon and blackness. That slice of blue opening to the shining light of the sun. The light after the storm before darkness descends…an answered prayer!

There was a knock on the door to our apartment. Fall 1977. I opened the door, and there stood…an angel! She looked familiar, I knew I recognized her, but couldn't place the name.

"Oh yea, you don't remember me, do you?"

"Nancy, right?" "You're my Dad's girlfriends cousin right?"

"I saw your dad and Jane over at the Weis Market a few minutes ago, and he told me to stop by to say Hi. They will be here in a minute."

"Please come in."

In that moment…that sliver of space and time between the horizon and the black emptiness of the sky, a slice of blue appeared and the sun broke through. I met another angel. I met the woman who would become my wife…the woman who would fulfill my life.

As fate and prayer would have it on that wonderful day in 1977 my pop's second wife introduced me to her cousin, Nancy Loraine Herr Boyd.

The bible records in Joel 2:25 that the Lord said "And I will restore to you the years that the locusts have eaten." Meeting Nancy, falling in love, marrying and having a family has provided me a joy and peace that passes understanding. I am complete.

A miracle? I believe. Over 35 years later, life is great again, but the center of the Universe is not me or even my lovely wife…The Author of Miracles who restored the years of destruction is on the throne of my life, and He is the center of the Universe.

Turns out Mom was right, "Everything will be ok." I love you mom…and I miss you. You'd really love Nance! She is almost as awesome as you!

Representative Scott Boyd is serving in his 5th term as a legislator in the PA House of Representatives. The Lancaster County native approaches public service in the Jeffersonian model as a "yeoman farmer". Losing his mother to breast cancer has been one of the most formative experiences of his life. Motivated by the grace of God in his life and the love of his wife and family, the former business owner serves the people of the 43rd legislative district with a passion and zeal for the traditional values central to the foundation of his legislative district.

Rom 8:19

Funny Moments and Smiles
Michelle Bruzzese

Moment 1. I'm a high school teacher. Early on I decided to tell my students about my diagnosis so they knew right from the start where I stood. I had my friend and co-worker in the room with me during my conversations with my three classes. Although I had practiced what I would say in advance, I found myself saying "Mrs. Francis will keep you abreast of the situation". She and I just looked at each other after those words and started cracking amid the tears that were falling from my face. The kids realized early on that we were both going to have a sense of humor about a tough topic and it helped to break their speechlessness and it let to good questions from them.

Moment 2. I worked during chemo so one day as the end of the school year neared I was just ready for it to end (I felt like you're lucky I'm here people). The same Mrs. Francis from above saw me walk through the door and said "Okay, I know you're my friend and all, and I know you have cancer but I just can't let you do this. You can't walk around wearing Crocs with socks! You just can't do it! I have to draw the line here." Of course I asked a student who was so quiet and sweet and she said: "Uhm! Well....actually...uhm! you really should just...just take the socks off." My friend told my other colleagues and I still get reminded of my "Crocs with socks" look.

Moment 3. When I was first diagnosed my husband would ask me to do things and I would reply "F.U.I.H.C!" (F U ...I have cancer!) if I just didn't feel up to it. It became a running joke between the two of us and helped us through a tough time.

I don't know if in writing this translates to funny moments but to me, during my rollercoaster of emotions these were funny stories.

Smiles…I do have a story on the flip side of this but with knowledge gained from it. I went to the Jersey Shore with my family because my generous co-workers raised money to give us a getaway. We went and had a great time. We had been there two years in a row before because it is a happy place for my kids. At the time, my kids were 5 and 7. They are two daring little boys that love rollercoasters and things. When you are on the boardwalk at night, it is filled with joyseekers. This night was no exception. I kept seeing people look at me (hairless and eyebrowless) and they would wince (the looks were like: "Aww this poor mom is going on the rollercoaster for the last time. How sad!" Sprinkled among the wincing and sad faces I would see a random smile. At the first and second smile I was like: "Why is this person smiling at me so big?" "Is this person crazy?" It wasn't until the wincing lead me to break down in a wave of tears that I realized that the smilers had the knowledge I didn't. The smilers were sending me a message of hope and positive thoughts because they must've known that I needed that. Before this I had been doing my usual routine outings with people that know me and knew I was doing well. It was the strangers feeling sorry for me that brought me discomfort, so the bottom line is, share your story with your own words when possible, and to everyone else I would say: if you ever see people you might suspect have cancer, just flash them a smile--it really is the best thing you can do.

Michelle lives in Stroudsburg, PA with her husband, Matt and sons, Daniel and Jeremy. She is a teacher at Pocono Mountain. You can reach her at mbeducadora@gmail.com.

The Story of a Breast Cancer Survivor
Linda Byrne

My breast cancer journey began in the Spring of 2007. It
was during a routine gynecological appointment; the doctor found
a large lump and requested further testing. I wasn't alarmed due to
my history of being cystic. A biopsy revealed that indeed, I did
have cancer. My oncologist/surgeon did a lumpectomy on June 3,
2007. This was followed by radiation and an adjuvant therapy,
(herceptin injections). This treatment was possible because I was
diagnosed as having HER2+ breast cancer.

There are many varieties of cancer, HER2+ is very
aggressive. I did some research and discovered the reason this
cancer is called HER2+ is because there are two or more HER2
genes for every normal gene in my cells, an over expression.   The
HER2 gene is found in the DNA of a cell. The purpose of the
HER2 gene is to help normal cells grow. HER2 protein is found
on the surface of cancer cells, also referred to as a HER2 receptor.
These HER2 tumors tend to grow and spread -more quickly than
HER2- tumors.   After radiation I began a series of herceptin
injections. When I finished my herceptin treatments, I continued
taking tamoxifen which I still take daily. During my treatment my
doctor did try another medication. After blood tests were run, he
found that I was peri-menopausal, not postmenopausal. In order
for this drug to be successful, you must be postmenopausal. Back
on tamoxifen I went. My theory for life being: "If I didn't have bad
luck, I wouldn't have luck at all". But truthfully, there were some
rays of sunshine throughout this whole process. I didn't lose my
hair, met great doctors and nurses, I didn't require a total
mastectomy and I'm still here to tell my story.

Breast cancer was not my first experience with a life
altering medical condition. Twenty-six years before breast cancer
I had suffered a closed head injury. That trauma happened in the
prime of my life. I was a recent graduate of The Pennsylvania
State University, a newlywed, and I had recently secured a great
job with a major oil company. I was all ready to begin a new

chapter in my life. Instead, I was severely injured in a motor vehicle accident. Life has never been the same!

My major at Penn State was Human Development, specializing in Early Childhood. I ruled out teaching after I did a semester at Children's Hospital of Philadelphia as a Play Therapist. I worked in a toddler playroom on one of the floors of CHOP. It is funny, CHOP is located next door to The Hospital of The University of Pennsylvania, where I was being treated for a massive brain injury. I was comatose for about four months. Life is fickle. CHOP'S newsletter had a picture of me in the playroom working with a patient on cognitive skills as a Therapist. Who would have thought that I'd be fighting for my life three years later.

My practicum at CHOP was a deciding factor in a career switch to the business world. As a newlywed, I was trying to keep costs down. I downsized on my insurance cost and benefits. The changes were not effective until the Monday AFTER my horrific car accident. The accident happened with my husband and I sitting unrestrained in the back seat of a friends VW bug. The accident happened in Lancaster County. I went initially to Ephrata Hospital where my parents were told to come. A doctor told my Mom all she could do was pray for a miracle. I was immediately transferred to HUP. At this great hospital I was still in a sorry shape. In fact, I received "Last Rites" three different times. I received radiation in such high doses, and numerous tests, NO WONDER I HAVE CANCER.

Sometimes I have a hard time accepting the hand I've been dealt. I have a fused elbow, artificial hip, visual and cognitive impairments and to boot, I am now a cancer survivor. Because of my misfortune, it made me stronger than I ever thought I'd be.

I struggle on disability trying to pay everything. I feel my purpose for living is to resonate to breast cancer and traumatic brain injury patients to 'NEVER GIVE UP'. As a disabled woman who lost everything, I'm still picking up the pieces; hoping for a better tomorrow...

Linda lives in Upper Darby, PA.

Briefly Scared Witless
Bobbi Chard

I thought I knew all about cancer. I was a caregiver for three members of my immediate family all who battled cancer and who lost their battle years ago. I witnessed first-hand how cancer could turn your life upside—in fact, I felt a little guilty about being the sole survivor of my family. Then the unexpected happened – their story became my story.

On April 19, 2006 I was diagnosed with breast cancer. I will never forget the doctor's words: "I'm sorry, but you have cancer." He went on to talk about my cancer and the plan of treatment but the more he talked the farther away his voice became as if he was in a tunnel. I was in shock. I was terrified—everyone I had known with cancer had died. Many thoughts came racing into my mind at this time--"Am I going to die too? Why me? Do I deserve this?" Then "Did I cause it? Was it the fish, the dairy, the wine or meat or nothing I did at all? Just the luck of the draw?

A simple truth became clear to me over the next few months ---cancer happens – it has no favorites or "target" groups – no age restraints or hunt for weakened victims. It strikes without preference, without warning and without reason.

I was overwhelmed by the people who had touched my life and expressed their love and support by sending me many cards, baskets of flowers, food, prayer and well wishes. I finally realized that there are so many great things about life and that God had work for me to do. But first, I needed to be strengthened and refined by personally going through this trial, not as a caregiver but as a patient. I fought very hard and focused on getting well.

I can praise God that He gave my husband, Dave the quiet courage, confidence, and strength needed to see us through this --- one of the worst times of our lives. He witnessed my immediate family members losing their battle with cancer and he lost his own brother to melanoma—a particular deadly type of skin cancer. Many people give in to fear and panic when they are presented with difficulties and at that time we were no exception. We were both scared witless.

But slowly and with great clarity I began to see things differently, as though the lens of the camera had been changed – everything looked brighter, cleaner, more colorful, more beautiful, and more precious. I realized that there are so many incredible things about life and that God had work for me to do. He strengthened Dave and me to endure and gave us what we needed to travel through our own journey with cancer.

After my surgery and treatment, I found help and support through the Breast Cancer Support Group at Mt. Nittany Medical Center. Dave drove me to the hospital to my first meeting, and said he would pick me up after the meeting was over. Close to the ending time of the meeting we heard a knock on the door of the meeting room and all the women who were attending the meeting stopped and looked over at the door – and there standing in the doorway was Dave – he came in and closed the door and said "May I stay? Breast cancer didn't happen to just Bobbi – it happened to both of us." I never loved him more than that moment when my sweet darling husband stepped out of his "comfort zone" to learn, support and comfort me.

I have been changed by cancer. I will never be the same again – physically, emotionally or spiritually. I realize that tomorrow is always uncertain, but each time I hug my husband or my sons and daughter and hold and love my grandchildren, I whisper a quiet prayer of thanks to God, who has helped us through it all. I am filled with gratitude for this time that I have been given.

In April I celebrated my five year anniversary of being "cancer free." I am a new person, able to respond to life's challenges with a spirit of "I can"--- and to claim myself a "victor" not a "victim" of one of life's most difficult challenge.

Bobbi lives in Pleasant Gap, PA, with her beloved husband, Dave. Together they enjoy four children and nine grandchildren. Bobbi and Dave share a clown/music ministry spreading the Word of

God through song, mime and clowning. Bobbi and Dave are retired and are enjoying their "golden" times together. They are members of "Happy Valley Alley" clown organization in State College. Dave is also director of the Paul Carney Banjo Band in State College.

A Sprinkle of FUN from Tammy…
Martha's Way or My Way…

Martha's Way: To keep potatoes from budding, place an apple in the bag with the potatoes.

My Way: Buy Instant Mashed Potatoes. They'll keep it in the pantry for well over a year.

Pushing to Do More
Dana Chestney

I had found a large lump in my breast while on a golf trip in April of 2007, however I kept it to myself. My son was in London as an exchange student and I wanted to make sure he was home safe before I made a doctor's appointment. When I found the lump I knew then that I had breast cancer. I had gone 7 years without a mammogram. He returned to PA in May of 2007.   I spent a happy week with him and decided it was time to call for a doctor's appointment. I was diagnosed in May 2007 at the age of 52.

I never once hesitated and I called Hershey Medical Center immediately for an appointment. I had invasive lobular breast cancer on my left side, tumor approximately 2 1/2 " x 2"1/2" x 2" deep into my chest. From the very beginning I decided to have a bilateral mastectomy, I knew I never wanted to go through treatment or news like this again.

I had chemo treatments first, July through November, mastectomy on November 12, 2007. During the operation I had a lung collapse and was put into intensive care for several days, which was a blessing. If this would not have happened, I would have been sent home the very next day.

Two weeks later, on Friday, November 23, 2007 I had to return to Hershey Medical Center to have a second operation and have additional surgery. By then my biopsy results were back and I still had cancer in 5 out of 7 lymph nodes. In January, I started on a pill form of chemo for 3 treatments, each treatment lasting 3 weeks, and 1 week rest. I then had a 2 week break and had 35 radiation treatments.

I told myself from the very beginning that I would beat this. I had a son who I wanted to see graduate from PSU in May 2008. My next goal was to see my daughter graduate in May 2009. I made small goals and would move from one to the next on.

I worked full time at Penn State Altoona during my chemotherapy treatments. I would travel to Hershey on Thursdays, working until noon, leave Altoona, and travel to Hershey for my

4pm appointment for chemo. I would work on Fridays, sometimes with a great struggle and then rest on the weekends.

It was April of 2008 that I attended a "Girls Night Out" event in Johnstown, PA, and I met Taunia Oshelin. I was so impressed with her story and battle of cancer that I approached her and volunteered to be on her committee if she ever brought "Girls Night Out" to Altoona. So began our annual "Girls Night Out" that we hold every October at the Jaffa Mosque in Altoona. My goal is for a cure to be found for this terrible disease.

Taunia has since passed away due to breast cancer; however, her program becomes larger and larger every year. The money raised in Altoona is split between the Joyce Murtha Breast Care Center and the Milton S. Hershey Medical Center. The Joyce Murtha Breast Care Center uses the money to fund free mammograms, and Hershey uses the funds to help find a cure.

I have a phenomenal relationship with the Hershey Medical Center. I have taken something negative and made a positive out of it. I have volunteered to work "Alex's Lemonade Stands" for neuro plasma cancer; have donated over $33,000 in the past two years to Hershey for a CURE, and just this past year I became the advisor for THON (Penn State Dance Marathon) at Penn State Altoona. Altoona was first place for the first time ever of all Commonwealth Campus locations and raised $97,228. Our highest amount ever at Altoona was $70,105 in 2009. I would have never become involved in finding a CURE for cancer if this hadn't affected me and my life. Now I try to do more and more.

Throughout it all, I truly believe that a POSITIVE ATTITUDE means everything!

Here are two notes that my friends wrote about me while battling cancer. Friends are very, very important. I wouldn't have been able to get through this without them. Written by Linda Filby, and Loane Maier

Becoming a Message Therapist for the Cause – Linda Filby

I'll never forget the day Loane and I became message therapists without any prior training, degree, or certificate. You know that Nike logo: 'Just Do It' well we just did it because it needed to be done. Our friend Dana had such severe reactions to her chemo treatment for bilateral breast cancer that she was crying due to the severe pain in her extremities. The tag team of Loane and Linda took each foot in hand and started rubbing and massaging Dana's feet and legs in our feeble attempt to give her comfort. We would have done anything she asked of us during those days. We liked to think it helped.

Golf Attire for Bald Women - Loane Maier

Why can't a woman just wear a ball cap or hat when playing golf during recovery from treatment from breast cancer? Dana can. She attempted to make everyone else comfortable with her bald head by covering it with a beautiful silk scarf and a hat for golf. It was so hot that day that she took off the scarf, at this point not caring what anyone thought, and just wore her hat. I was very proud of her that day, she was beautiful. She worked very hard during treatment, losing her lovely locks as a side effect. But she got some happy, carefree therapy that day with her friends playing golf. We didn't even keep our golf scores; we scored without numbers just being together.

Dana Chestney lives in Altoona, PA with her husband Jeff of 35 years. She is employed by Penn State University and works in the admissions office at Penn State Altoona. You can reach Dana at ddc3@psu.edu.

Disguised Blessing
Judy Clouser

My story started when I was having a breast reduction surgery due to back problems. It was discovered that I had a Stage 3 cancer in one of my breasts.

Two days after the stitches were removed from the surgery, I had a mastectomy and 27 lymph nodes were removed from under my arm.

After one year, I under went a breast rebuilding, using a flap from my stomach. It took 2 years to heal completely. I do not recommend it!

I have a message for large breasted women, prior to the reduction I was a 44 DD. The mammogram was completely negative before this surgery. I was fibrous, but not one sign of cancer! If not for the reduction they say I would have died due to the cancer.

I thank Jesus for his guiding me to the reduction!

Tammy asked me to consider a few questions for this piece:

What did you learn through this process? I didn't go through the surgery alone. Jesus was with me.

What words of encouragement could you offer others? Have a positive attitude, KNOW that you will be well!

Is there anything you wish you knew before going through this? I wish I had known how sick I was going to be with the chemo.

Is there anything you wish your doctor would have told you? How painful the stomach flap removal was going to be.

Can you identify anything humorous that happened on this path to recovery? I learned to cover my bald head when it rained.

That was 11 years ago and I'm happy to say; God has brought me safely thru!

Judy is a 62 year old happily married for 42 years woman. Having been born and raised in Michigan, she has lived her entire life in the state. She loves spending time with her husband, her daughter, and son, and their family's. Her special joy is her grandchildren: 19, 18, 3 and 8 months.

A Sprinkle of FUN from Tammy…
Martha's Way or My Way

Martha's Way: Place a slice of apple in hardened brown sugar to soften it.

My Way: Brown sugar is supposed to be soft?

I Won't Let Go
Dianne Crust

In 1987 my mother, Baba, was diagnosed with breast cancer; in 1996 my sister Terri was diagnosed with breast cancer; in 2003 my mother's sister, (my favorite aunt) Patti was diagnosed with breast cancer, and in 2005 her daughter Karen was diagnosed with breast cancer. Through all their treatments, reconstructive surgeries and continued battles with cancer, my message to them was: "if I could fight this fight for you I would. I hate that you are going through this, and although there are days when you just want to give up…please keep fighting because I love you and can't live without you". Through the years, I've seen more family and friends face the struggles and hardships from this terrible disease. And I still have this overwhelming desire to let them know that they are very special to me, and I need them to fight this, because I can't let go.

Then one day in April, I was driving along and Rascal Flatts song *I Won't Let Go* came on the radio. I have a dear friend, Phyllis, who was just going through her chemo treatments at that time, and again I felt, "if I could fight this fight for you I would, but since I can't, please know that I'm here and I'll always be". I'm sure there isn't a caregiver, family member or friend who has a loved one facing this battle that doesn't "feel" the words to this song deep in their hearts and souls. I had to pull over and have a good cry…I went right out and got the CD and gave it to Phyllis to let her know she is very special to me.

So, to my Mom, my sister Terri, my Aunt Patti, my cousin Karen, my sister Bev, my dear friends Tammy and Dana… and to you Phyllis…please know "I Won't Let Go".

Dianne lives in Boalsburg, PA with her best friend and husband of 36 years, John. She is blessed with two beautiful daughters, Shelli and Paula, and a very handsome son-in-law Ryan. Her greatest gifts are her two precious granddaughters, Princess Madelyn and Princess Lily with the "triple crown" expected in January 2012.

Running the Show
Allison Cummings

On June 15th 2010 at 2:47 pm, I received the call from my breast surgeon telling me that I had early stage-one breast cancer at the age of 39. Who has to worry about breast cancer at that age? I soon found out women 10-15 years younger than me worried about breast cancer. When my surgeon called, I was standing by my bedroom closet. When I hung up the phone, I called my family and then sat there crying my eyes out for about ten minutes.

I decided that while I have breast cancer, it would never have me. I would run the show and cancer would never dictate a moment of my life going forward. I have never asked "why me?" Why not me? It is not like I had a big neon sign over my head saying "no cancer allowed here".

I do have a new "normal" since my diagnosis. I am still the same person but don't let the little things get to me anymore. I don't allow toxic people in my life. Fellow survivors had told me, that once you start telling friends about your diagnosis that you will quickly learn who your real friends are. I like to say that it quickly separated the men from the boys.

I have to constantly remind myself to slow down. I work out on a regular basis and I ate decently before diagnosis. Post diagnosis I work on becoming very attuned to my body and what are the best foods to fuel it. I read labels, I drink more water, and I pay attention to food and nutrition studies. I have added strength training to my workout regimen because it is important to keep my strength, balance, and bone density.

I wrote a book about my experience for my nephew who is three. It is very important to me that he knows how strong his auntie was in beating breast cancer. I want to show women that you can get through a breast cancer diagnosis and treatment and thrive.

To whom much is given, much is expected

Allison lives in Austin TX with her spoiled shih-tzu Shelby. She works with families going through crisis and you can reach her at http://www.facebook.com/alli3300.

A Sprinkle of FUN from Tammy…

"I never married because there was no need. I have three pets at home who answer the same purpose as a husband. I have a dog that growls every morning, a parrot that swears all afternoon, and a cat that comes home late every night."

-- Marie Corelli

A Pink Ribbon Story
Dedicated to
Sharon Dapp

Despite the fact that cancer hits you hard, and hits you suddenly, life must go on and this was Sharon Dapp's main inspiration as she challenged herself to keep things as normal as possible in her life.

It was in August of 2005 when Sharon discovered she had breast cancer. And it was by no mishap. At the time, she was accompanying her daughter, Selena, for support to the Breast Health Center in Williamsport, Pennsylvania.

Previously, Selena had been screened for a lump in her breast, and was scheduled to have it removed. In the meantime, Sharon had a routine mammogram that revealed an abnormal mass in her right breast. Both women were scheduled for surgery the same day.

Fortunately, for Salena, hers turned out to be a benign cyst, whereas, Sharon's biopsy was diagnosed with the beginning stages of cancer. She was only 49. Selena got to go home that day after her surgery, but Sharon did not. She remained for further testing and surgery was scheduled shortly afterwards to remove a large mass from Sharon's breast. It looked like a "big splatter." She was able to go home the same day as the scheduled surgery, and a few days later Sharon went back to the hospital for radiation treatments.

Throughout the remaining days, family and friends said she remained strong and calm. Sharon had to endure 50 radiation treatments, and she would go every day after work Monday through Friday for about 8 weeks.

Co-workers said she was exhausted but she wanted to still work everyday working at a small newspaper office as the office manager. "Yes I was here when she had breast cancer.... so sad, but she was determined to fight and be strong and that she was! , said Crystal Shrawder from Hughesville and one or her assistants. "She handled her treatments so very well, it was amazing!"

Although she was extremely tired, Sharon felt she needed to work as they were short on help as it was, and it made her feel needed. She had been employed with the company since she was 18.

On the last day of her radiation treatment, she and her best friend, Linda Neupauer, celebrated. Every year when her birthday comes around on March 8, Sharon celebrates being a survivor. "I beat it, and no chemo was needed" she said, and every year that goes by without detection is a blessing for her. "I regret I can't give blood anymore. I was a regular donor up until the cancer," she said.

"On the day of her last radiation treatment in October, she wanted to go shopping at the Reading Outlets," replied her best friend, Linda. And to this day, the twosome still take an annual three day shopping trip every October to celebrate being a survivor.

Sharon Dapp
As written by Barbara C. Barrett

Sharon Dapp lives in Montoursville, PA with her husband Andy. She loves to shop with her best friend and visit the casinos when they have time.

A Sprinkle of FUN from Tammy…

"I'm not offended by all the dumb blonde jokes because I know I'm not dumb and I certainly know I'm not blonde." -- Dolly Parton

A Turkey Baster?
Marian Davis

It all started fourteen years ago. At the time I knew absolutely no one who had breast cancer, but I was about to learn about it and real fast!

In January of that year I had a mammogram and a visit to the doctor to check for polyps. The mammogram was clear and the doctor just wanted to see me in a few months to check on the polyps again. About nine months later I received a card to make an appointment and while I was there the doctor decided to give me a check-up, even though it wasn't time for the yearly mammogram yet.

During the exam, he detected a lump. He checked the mammogram and verified that it had not been there just nine months earlier. So began my education and experience with breast cancer.

I did not want to read about people with breast cancer, but I wanted to talk with someone. Personally, I needed the face to face to be able to ask questions and have a better understanding about what was happening and what was going to happen in my near future. What I really wanted was for someone to tell me it was going to be okay.

Fortunately, I was able to find a very good support group in my area and they provided some answers and support that I needed.

I went through the necessary surgery and came home with a drain in place. Even though my daughter is a physician's assistant, I still didn't know a lot about a drain. I understood that a drain was in place so that something could "drain", that made sense. Over the weekend, I had a visiting nurse stop by to check on my progress. When she got there, she told me there was a blockage and she had to get something to unplug the blockage. We both thought about it for a minute when it suddenly hit me – a turkey baster! Maybe now would be a good time to tell you that I try very hard to find the humor in everything in life! There are a lot of serious things that happen in life but you must stay positive and look for the humor.

We both laughed about the turkey baster, and although she said it would work perfectly for the job at hand, she opted to use a syringe instead. Too late, we may have used a syringe, but I have never looked at a turkey baster the same way again, and maybe after reading this story, you won't either! I shared this story with my support group and we had a great laugh, at least for most of us.

Going through chemo gave me some added challenges. Personally, I could have done without them! One of the added challenges was weight gain. I started to go to Weight Watchers and one night a woman came up to me and asked if I was in the local breast cancer support group. I told her I was and she said she recognized me. She proceeded to tell me that she heard my turkey baster story and was absolutely appalled that I could make fun of such a serious matter. I told her I certainly didn't mean to offend anyone but I was telling the story about my own experience. She was still upset, but it served as a reminder to me that we all look at things differently. I hope one day she will recognize the great value of laughter, especially when that laughter is about yourself and even when it revolves around a very serious issue.

Although a cancer diagnosis is very serious, there were a lot of funny things that happened along the way. One day my granddaughter came to see me and I needed a bathing suit. We went shopping and we had a very good, healthy laugh when we discussed how I was going to find just the right bathing suit with one "boob" bigger than the other one! I couldn't change what was happening, but I wasn't going to let it get me down and "win" either.

My life is full of strange circumstances. The way the doctor found this lump before my regularly scheduled exam and it wasn't there before was very strange indeed, but it wasn't the only example of such incidents. For example, sometime ago my brother passed away. On the long drive to his memorial service I felt like my sciatic nerve was pinched and I had a lot of pain. It didn't seem to want to go away so I finally called the doctor to see about having the nerve checked. When he checked things out and ultimately did an ultrasound, he found that I had bladder cancer.

In June of this year I thought I had the flu. I just couldn't get over it no matter what I tried. The doctor checked my stomach and found that I have something else going on in there. Had it not been for the polyps we wouldn't have found breast cancer; if not for the sciatic nerve we wouldn't have found bladder cancer, and if not for..., well, you get the idea! It seems as though all things in life come together for a purpose.

I wanted to make sure the cancer was gone and went to added lengths to make sure that happened. I opted for a longer period of chemo to have a better chance of getting everything nasty out of my system. During my chemo, I was having some very bad reactions, including tremendous mouth sores, to the point that I couldn't even open my mouth. My doctor was out of town but he called to see how I was doing. When I told him about the mouth sores, he called in a prescription. The rinse he prescribed seemed to make matters worse before they got better and the first night I used it was one of the worst nights I had throughout the entire ordeal.

Your opinion of what I am about to state here is your opinion, but I can tell you it is the honest to goodness truth. The first night of the rinse I was so sick and miserable and I just didn't think I could go on any longer. After all this time, it was the first night that I had cried. My husband was very helpful and I had to crawl up the stairs. He left for work before I awoke. When I did wake up at 10 AM, I found myself alone in the house and in tremendous pain and miserable. I prayed and prayed that the Lord would help me get through this. At that very moment, I heard my name being called, very plainly and there was no mistaking who was calling, it was Momma. Momma was what some people would call a "good Presbyterian woman". She was a woman of tremendous faith. A mother calling a daughter's name isn't anything out of the ordinary, except that my dear mother had passed away in 1993! You can believe what you will but I heard her as plain as if she were sitting beside me. She called my name

92

three times, very clearly. That was a turning point in my recovery path and from there I felt like a weight had been lifted from my shoulders and I was on my way to recovery!

I was interested in sharing my story here because I hope this story, and the others in this book will help people understand that they will get through difficult times in life. I encourage people to find a good support group in their area, or at least have a strong support group of family and friends. Often it is easier to talk it out, and sometimes easier with people who are compassionate and understand, but not necessarily your family.

Breast cancer has certainly made me more compassionate and hopefully more thoughtful of others. Some say it is a gift and I would agree. For me, breast cancer helped put things into perspective in my life. I have always had a strong faith, but my experience with breast cancer helped to cement my faith. I know there are some people who live their lives without faith. I just don't know how they do it and I feel very blessed to know that the Lord is indeed in control.

Marian Davis
As written by Tammy Miller

Marian is from Meadville, PA and was a very busy business owner and mother of three for years. She is now a very busy retired mother of three and grandmother of four. She is actively involved along with her husband, with their grandchildren, church work and community. And happily involved—she is quick to add.

My Celebration Party
Heidi Eck

The tent was set up, the centerpieces were made, and friends had made all kinds of appetizers, finger sandwiches and desserts. The coolers were filled with all types of drinks. I had made a special pink punch and even got the fancy punch bowl out to serve it. My friends and I had made favors for everyone. It wasn't the nicest day outside, but it didn't matter. It was my Celebration of Life party - I was celebrating 5 years cancer free. I sent out the most awesome photo invitations with a good picture of my son and me. I invited over 100 people and 93 were able to stop by. It was a drop in hosted by my son, 6 years old at the time and me. The reason for the party started five years prior......

From the time I was 31 years old, I went for mammograms and ultrasounds for keeping a check on fibroid cysts. October 1, 2004, was the beginning of Breast Cancer Awareness month, I noticed as I walked into the facility for my annual tests. When I left that day, I was one of those women who were in utter shock that I could possibly have breast cancer. I was only 36! I had a husband of 12 years and a 19 month old son. I didn't have time for this! It really was going to be a bump in the road of life! Little did I know the little miracles I would encounter on my cancer treatment journey.

My friend and pastor Mary Ellen made a commitment to come to every appointment and test. She was a great source of strength and humor. She took me to get a short haircut before I started chemotherapy. She also took me to each chemo treatment and brought me Reese's Peanut Butter cups and celery with peanut butter.

My most memorable memory was when I was taken to the OR early for my surgery and Mary Ellen hadn't met us in the pre-op room. The phone rang as the surgeon, anesthesiologist and nurses were preparing. The surgeon informed me that we would have to wait to start because my "minister" was on her way down. She showed up a few minutes later, in surgical scrubs and a mask-

94

it was the only way that would let her in to pray with me. The anesthesiologist reminded her not to touch my hand that already had the IV line in it. She said, "let us bow our heads" and everyone in the OR bowed and said "Amen" when she was finished. Doesn't get much better than that to have your surgical team pray with you!

The amount of people who volunteered to help out my family and me was just overwhelming. There was my best friend, Karen, who did the wash and babysat the week after chemo, my father-in-law who came down every morning to make breakfast, my mom who babysat in the afternoons, friends who coordinated the meals through all the schools at which I worked. There were the meal makers, babysitters, Christmas present wrappers, washers and just general helpers. I think one of the most important things to remember is that when you go through cancer treatment, you must let other people help you.

Did you know that everything now comes in pink? It does and I own it. I have pink kitchen utensils, pink candles, every pink breast Christmas tree ornament known to man….you get the picture. What I did understand was that every time someone saw something that referred to the pink ribbon or breast cancer, they thought of me and my battle with cancer, and that was the thought behind the purchase. While it is humorous sometimes, it is very thoughtful.

What was most helpful in my journey through cancer treatment was the support from "mentors" as I called them. Sometimes a friend would tell a friend who was a fellow survivor. Then that person would call me. It was the most comforting thing to talk to someone who was on the other side of treatment and survived! One key person was an 11 year survivor at the time. She told me to ask her anything. That is truly the way to find out exactly what is going to happen with surgery, chemo, radiation and oral hormone therapy. I always call people as soon as someone tells me he/she has a friend or relative with cancer. I want to make sure I help others who are newly diagnosed as I was helped.

Some of the most monumental memories deal with my son. He decided during a church service one time to pull the wig off of my head. Once he could say wig he would tell people in the grocery store that his mommy had a wig and it would come off. One night I came in his bedroom to find the wig on the dancing boobah that he got for his birthday....you never know where the wig was going to show up.

My goal for the end of chemotherapy was a trip to Disney World. I eventually got to that goal. There were little goals to have along the way. Like a "halfway through chemo" dinner out, an Easter trip to Vermont and a Mother's Day trip to the Hershey Hotel Brunch. I am so glad I took time to celebrate the monumental milestones in a journey I had no idea I was taking!

The cancer treatment plan for me was not a short one. It was 1 ½ years until I was done with chemotherapy. I was one of the fortunate survivors who was able to receive herceptin and am able to take arimidex.

One thing I have learned from cancer is how not to worry about the little things in life. I have a joke with some of my friends at work and my current boss - if people really want to get upset, let me show them the scars........seriously. When we think about what we go through to live our lives, do the little things that upset us really mean much?

You can survive the words "you have cancer". You can survive the treatment. You just have to make up your mind and you can do what you have to do to get through treatment. There are so many angels that will help you along the way!

Heidi lives in Myerstown, PA with her 8 year old son Jeremy. She is an elementary music teacher, cub scout leader and a soccer mom. She loves traveling, scrapbooking and entertaining family and friends.

Coming or Going
Barbara Eyrich

Breast Cancer….not the words you want to hear from your doctor. You have choices when you hear these words; the first is to let it sink in, the next to make your plan of attack and go with it.

My Mom and sister are both breast cancer survivors and so it was always in the back of my mind when my annual mammogram was done….is this the year I get my diagnosis. Well, that came in May of 2010. I had gone in for my routine mammogram and received a call that I needed to go back for another check…the dreaded extra compression mammogram. For anyone that has not had this done, they flatten you even more than they do with a regular mammo. Once this is completed, they have you wait while a doctor looks at it right away. A nurse came out and called my name…I knew what that meant; I had to go for further testing. They took me back into a room where I now had to have an ultrasound done of my breast. Unfortunately, this showed a lump. The doctor explained that I would need to have a biopsy done in order to determine if it was cancer or not. She went over the options and we scheduled an appointment.

I went for the biopsy and then got the dreaded call...."Mrs. Eyrich, you have breast cancer". Unfortunately for me, once I heard those words everything else was a blur. I remember sitting in my office with the door closed crying uncontrollably because I didn't want it to be me that was dealing with this. Once I mustered up the strength to stop crying I phoned my husband Jim to give him the bad news. As I was trying to sound audible to him he did manage to hear "cancer" and tried to console me. He was my rock; he gave me the strength I needed at that time to calm myself down and face the reality that we needed to be as prepared and focused as possible to make the best of this situation.

We met with the surgeon to discuss my options and schedule surgery. He was optimistic that since we caught this early (my lump was 1.5 cm) that I would most likely just need the surgery and lymph node dissection and then radiation after I healed. The day came and my husband and I went to the hospital for the AM surgery. I was not so lucky though, I woke up very late that night with a drain in. As soon as I saw it I knew the cancer had traveled into my lymph system and chemo was now going to be a part of my treatment. I started to cry right away with my husband trying to comfort me.

Family....what can I say about family? My family is wonderful. They were a great resource for me as I started on this journey. My husband and I are blessed with three great kids two of which are married. We also have three grandkids which helped to keep me focused on the end result....getting through all of the tests and treatments needed to make me healthy again. My siblings were also a great resource for me. Whether it was to call them up and vent my frustrations and fears or to cry; they always listened and knew what to say to help me get through whatever it was at that time.

Chemo was not something I looked forward to facing, however I knew it was what was best for me. My doctor suggested that since I was young (49) and was in pretty good physical shape she would go as aggressive as she could with the drugs and as often as was allowable to hit this hard. I was very fortunate to have someone drive me to and from chemo every other week and for my follow up injection the day after. You never know how many true friends you have until facing something like this. They are what helped to make this journey a little easier to travel. I was also fortunate that I only had to have one treatment, my last one, to be postponed due to a low count.

Once the chemo started I was watching my hair all the time. I knew with the drugs I was going to be on that the hair was definitely going to fall out. I had made a conscious decision to take control of that in the hopes that it would be easier to face. Boy was I wrong! As my husband was shaving my head with my daughter looking on, I was a mess. I was bawling uncontrollably. It was very difficult to look at myself in the mirror and honestly I think it was a month later before I took a really good look at myself. I opted to wear scarves not a wig. I did buy a wig, however I did not like the way it felt at all on my head. I was not sure how I would be for the holidays. I had already told the kids that they should just go ahead and make plans that we would be okay. What a pleasant surprise when I received a call from our daughter stating they would have Thanksgiving at our house if I was okay with that. They made everything and we had the best Thanksgiving I could ever ask for. My chemo ended on December 13th, three days before my 50th birthday and 12 days before Christmas. By Christmas I was feeling stronger each day with minor limitations. What a great way to end the year…what more could I ask for?

Radiation was a piece of cake. The girls were so nice that I met with every day. They were always upbeat and cheery. The last day I decided I needed to do something so I had my husband write on my breast "thank you ☺". The girls loved it. As I explained to them, they saw my breast for the last 29 days I figured I needed to do something to break up the monotony.

All throughout this process; once I had gotten over all of the "firsts" I realized that I needed to keep my sense of humor. I remember around Halloween, we were sitting at the dinner table and my husband started to laugh. When my daughter and I looked at him with a puzzled look, he said "I think we should paint your head orange". I asked why and he said then we can draw a face on it and you will have a pumpkin head. Then my daughter said, "How about we paint a face on the back of your head…then we won't know if you are coming or going".

When my hair started to grow, my husband said, "You remind me of a Chia pet". We laughed really hard!! I was so excited one day when I got up because my hair (what I had of it) had been kind of matted to my head. I actually had "bed head" and I was happy about it.

Barb is 50 years old and married to a great guy, Jim. They have three wonderful kids -- Chris and his wife Rachel, Jess and her husband Paul and Jamie and her fiancé Brandon. They also have three awesome grandkids -- Logan, Mason and Madelyn. Barb is a Loan CSR for Harleysville Savings Bank, a job she thoroughly enjoys. She likes photography, being outdoors and going to the mountains.

A Sprinkle of FUN from Tammy...

A few weeks after my surgery, I went out to play catch with my golden retriever. When I bent over to pick up the ball, my prosthesis fell out. The dog snatched it, and I found myself chasing him down the road yelling "Hey, come back here with my breast!" -- Linda Ellerbee

Strength Through Animals
Theresa Farabaugh

I was diagnosed with breast cancer on March 12, 2010. I have three dogs, one I just adopted a few months before my diagnosis, and I was so scared that I was going to die, and leave my dogs without someone to love and walk with them. I know my husband would care for them, but not to the detail that I would, and I felt guilty for adopting Angel, a Lab/Pit Bull mix, for fear that I would not be around to raise her.

After a year of many doctor appointments, surgery, chemo, and sickness, I am here to say that the best thing I could have done was to adopt that pup named Angel. I tried to walk my three dogs every day that I could, even when I felt like I had no strength in me. I had Angel and Junie (my Husky who was seven years old), on the same leash. Junie wanted to just go, go, go, like she always does, not realizing that I could not. I would stop often to cool off and that would help me to continue. Junie did not want to stop, she would keep pulling on the leash, Angel took care of her. Angel would just sit down and would not let Junie pull me until I said let's go. Only then would Angel stand and start to walk. Angel would pull back on the leash to tell Junie to slow down. How that pup knew what was going on with me I will never know.

I have since trained her to not run away from me and to come back when called. I live on a farm, where I walk and can let Angel and Sandy run freely. They listen well. I got both of them as pups. Junie, the Husky, will run away the first chance she gets.

Finally, there is Sandy. She is a Lab, Husky mix and is six years old. She loves to hunt for anything the farm has to offer, especially groundhogs. She usually runs ahead of me to scout the field for her prey. When I would receive chemo, she would not leave my side when we walked. She would not go out hunting. The second and third week after chemo when I was feeling better, she would venture a little further and hunt. The week I received chemo again, she was by my side to stay. The year I was receiving chemo treatments, Sandy only got 17 groundhogs, but the year

101

before she got 34. She is a faithful friend. So far this year she has only gotten two groundhogs, but the year is young.

One day Junie got away from me and she took off running, Sandy running after her. When I got to the top of the hill, there was Junie and Sandy sitting and waiting for me. I heard Sandy barking at Junie, so I guess Sandy told Junie to behave, and wait for me.

After my last chemo treatment I was depressed and weak and did not know if I was going to keep on living. One night I decided to pull weeds in my garden. As I knelt there praying, pulling weeds and crying, who appeared beside me but Angel? She started licking my tears away, as if to say I am here for you. We have a two foot fence around the garden and she had never been in my garden before or since. That day she knew I needed strength to keep on going.

One year later I realized I was blessed to get Angel, who was truly an "angel" when I needed her most. I walk with my dogs every chance I get. On days that I do not feel like walking, whether it was during chemo or now, my three girls give me the devil and make me feel guilty. All three of them will start howling, whining, and barking. They sound like I am being violent with them. The neighbors now realize I came home from work and it is just time for me to walk the dogs.

I thank you for all that you are doing. I hope every "breast buddy" knows there is life before, during, and after breast cancer. You have to look for the strength from God and His creatures to keep you going.

Theresa lives on a farm in Ebensburg, PA with her husband Jim, and of course, her three dogs, Junie, Angel and Sandy. She works as a Medical Assistant at the Altoona Arthritis and Osteoporosis Center.

He Prays
Sarah Farrugia

I hate it when he prays. Really. I hate it. It offends me that he spends so much time praying to these icons around our house, turning on all the lights so that, in his words, he is praying to God in light and honouring the presence of the Lord. It's offensive to me. Offensive you see because the more he prays, the sicker I get. Sicker and sicker and sicker. Weaker and weaker and weaker. My body is riddled, my mind is chaotic and my spirit, well my spirit is broken. I am broken. And he, he seems to think that by praying, things will be ok. God will look after us ... apparently but I don't see it his way. Show me proof. Where is the proof that God loves us and cares for us? Cares for me?

Where was God when I was diagnosed with this horrible cancer? This horrid disease that walks with you, beside you every single day of your life. I thought God walked beside us all, protecting us, loving us, caring for us. What happened? Did the cancer say to God 'get out of the way, I will walk beside this person now. I will haunt her for the rest of her days. Scans may come up clear when I've lost focus for an hour or two, but I'm always there, always with her. Medical biopsies and mammograms may come up clear one month, then suspect the next. She will never rest. I'll make sure that she lives out her days with a dark storm cloud hanging over her head'. And what did God do? Did God even put up a fight? Did God even try to fight the cancer saying 'no, she is a good person? She is kind and caring and honest. She is loyal to family and friends. She who you are trying to destroy is not deserving of this fate. Get the hell out of my way cancer, I God, walk beside her?' Well, were you there God? Did you put up a fight, or did you fall back on being the 'All Peaceful' and just give in and agree to move over to let cancer walk beside me? Well? Answer me.

But he, he prays. Every morning and every night. He prays and prays and worships and prays. He kisses the bright red book with the words 'Holy Bible' boldly printed on the cover.

Bold and arrogantly printed in gold lettering. The red dust jacket is tattered and torn through much handling. He believes and prays, each day. And he must not be interrupted. All lights blazing and every scrap of paper, iconic picture or pamphlet ever picked up from a Church must be laid out, face up as offerings to God. Printed pictures of revered paintings of St. Christopher, the Virgin Mary, Jesus and St. Francis, creased and torn, are all laid out. The tacky clock depicting Jesus and his apostles at The Last Supper, his golden chain with the charm of yet another Virgin Mary, an old mass book with a softened leather cover and old Rosary Beads which once belonged to his great, great grandmother are all laid out. And for an hour he prays. He prays and I become angrier and angrier and weaker and weaker. He kisses the icon pictures, the gold chain, the Rosary, the mass book and the arrogant red book. I hear the kisses. He kisses them out of respect for God he tells me. I seethe. He knows that I seethe. He believes. He despises my cynicism. What do I care? I am the one carrying the burden. I seethe and he prays.

Did I tell you that my hair now is short and grey? I had it all cut off at the beginning of treatment. The nurses in oncology suggested this. They said my hair would fall out soon enough after my first session of chemotherapy. The trauma of losing it would be considerably diluted if my hair was already short. Easier to cope with. So, it all came off. My beautiful auburn hair. Straight and shiny. Long hair which fell down my back almost to the belt of my jeans. Long, healthy hair. My crowning glory. I took such good care of it. So healthy and lustrous. My hairdresser didn't even charge me for cutting it all off. I told her my situation and she cried with me. Fittingly she showed the required amount of emotion and with empathy she shaved off my crown. The auburn tresses which once fell down my back now fell down onto the parquetry floor. Shiny floor, shiny hair like some bizarre collage quickly and emotionlessly mixed in with the bottle blond split ends of the hair of the woman sitting next to me. She didn't look after her hair. The assistant came along with her broom and swept it all away. In the mirror I faced a woman I did not know. The stylists deft hand equipped with a man's shaver had delivered a foreign being with pained eyes and hideously short hair. He prayed for me that night. He prayed for me and for the remaining crop of hair on my head. He need not have bothered. The hair barely lasted the three weeks until my next dose of chemotherapy. No hair left now. Just a bald head on a woman even more hideous that before. I wore a sleeping cap to bed and showered in the dark so that no one including me would catch a glimpse of my naked, vulnerable, ugly head.

He prayed that the chemo would work. That the poison that coursed through my veins would stamp out the cancer, kill it and save my life. As I sat in the sterile room, attached to the drip I could smell the cocktail of chemicals and medication. The smell assaulted my nose and made me sick to the stomach. The blue liquid being delivered through the needle, into my hand and my vein made me feel a weird kind of sickness. I prayed too now. Prayed that I would fall asleep and not wake up.

Through all six sessions of chemotherapy followed by six weeks of radiation treatment my husband continued to pray to God that the treatment would work, that I would get better, that our lives would return to normal. I knew that this would not be the case. I knew my life would never be as it was. I was right.

Now 18 months out of treatment, I have had my fair share of scares and worries. Scans that have shown up with concerns requiring further follow up with biopsies. I still take my medication which slowly leaches my bones of calcium. I have been recently diagnosed with early onset osteoporosis. He keeps praying my husband. Every morning and every night. He prays for me, for himself, for our families and friends. For those who supported us through such horrific times. He even prays for those who let us down. When I take a moment to reflect on what has been I realise that I am both right and wrong.

I was wrong in begrudging his prayers and his faith. Each to their own. Everyone copes with life in their own way. He through Christianity and me, through my search of spirituality of a different kind; yoga and meditation. I was also right. My life, our lives would never be the same again. Cancer walks beside me every minute of every day but I am a survivor now, not a victim. I still wrestle with my demons of friendships lost and loyalties broken, but everyday I am amazed at his loyalty, both to God, to himself and to me. It would have been so easy for him to lose faith. He could have turned his back on me and walked away. So now, I too pray everyday. I pray for other cancer patients, I pray for the medical staff that care so much, and I pray for family and friends. Most of all though, I pray for my husband and thank God and Universe that he is He, and I am me and together we will move forward. Maybe the cancer came to me to teach me a lesson, to teach me that he is a good man and that all things happen for a reason.

Sarah lives in Melbourne, Australia with her wonderfully supportive husband Ray, Cosmo the cat and Baci the Beagle. She works for The Body Shop as a sales advisor and make-up artist whilst completing a Diploma of Professional Writing. She has been fortunate to meet some amazing people during her breast cancer treatment.

A Sprinkle of FUN from Tammy…

"My second favorite household chore is ironing; my first being hitting my head on the top bunk bed until I faint."

--Erma Bombeck

The Poetry of Breast Cancer
Cynthia Finch

"I could hear the blood singing in my veins," stuff of songwriters, poets, novelists. That's what it felt like when the lump was removed, the lymph nodes removed, things pretty much healed up, and I had to start radiation.

I remember how my heart sank when the oncologist told me I would be doing that. I didn't have chemo, so in that way I was lucky. It was only in the first stage. When they found it hadn't spread, I thought that would be it, no other treatment required. However, I was so sure that breast cancer was a death sentence that when it seemed not to be and I was getting up at 6 AM every morning to drive over to the hospital and have the radiation treatment, I found myself exhilarated.

Everyone told me I would be so tired I should take a futon mattress up to my office so I could rest; maybe take a leave of absence. (I was lucky to be teaching at a university, so I had some free days when I only needed to sit and grade or do reading for classes.) But I was full of energy, good will, big grins, delighted wonder that I was not dying. People reacted positively to my new demeanor, sometimes looking at me in amazement. I think there are some people in the world I call people of good will. They seem to radiate positive energy, kind of like, to name someone we may all know of, Will Smith in some of his funnier rolls. At that particular time, I was graced with some of that. While I couldn't talk the police officer out of a speeding ticket (I was late getting to the hospital that day), he told me it had been a "really great pleasure, Ma'am" talking to me. I guess the result of that encounter could have been better but it was more pleasant than surliness would have been.

There was a young man getting radiation for a tumor in his throat area. He and I would cheerfully chat as we waited for the treatment every morning. One day he wasn't there – I asked about him and found out that he had had a second opinion. They had sent the cancerous tissue to another lab which said it was in fact not cancerous. The radiation had damaged his salivary glands, so it was so good that he could stop. Don't you wonder how they can make such mistakes?

One thing I learned, though I didn't apply it to myself, was that sometimes it's more than good to get a second opinion.

Another thing I learned is that not all of us are good group people, although many people are helped by becoming part of a group to talk about our experiences and problems. I went to a talk and information session run by an oncologist new to this area. After he had talked, many women spoke up about problems they had had with their treatment, their doctors, anything related to having had breast cancer. It turned into what I would call a "whine meeting" – and as I found that unhelpful and even depressing, I never went to any other group meetings after that. I didn't miss them.

This doesn't mean that others don't get a lot out of them. A good friend and colleague had breast cancer after I did, and she was very active in groups, began to form them, ran them, conducted focus groups on how to help others, so this kind of group can be very beneficial to many women facing treatment and recovery. It is good to have a support system.

I found out that I personally do better if I don't concentrate on major problems like this one, and hear others' sad and terrible stories about their experiences. In fact, I don't even remember the exact year I went through this – I think it was 1993, though. Oddly, I remember the date – August third. I don't mean I believe people should just "forget about it" – even if not impossible, pretending it never happened wouldn't be helpful in the long run.

One thing I wish had been in place when I was going through this is the "sentinel node" operation to remove lymph nodes. They took a lot of mine, not just the one where the cancer would first have spread if it was going to. And as a result I have pretty bad lymphedema in one arm. But I just keep going anyway, and buy interesting elastic sleeves from a wild and creative company on the web.

Another dear friend of mine had breast cancer a few years after I did, and I told her about that sentinel node procedure. She had been worried as she liked to be very active, do a lot of work around the house, sports, etc., and was upset about perhaps not being able to do all that. She actually had to change doctors – her first one refused to do it. I don't know if this is still happening, but check it out if you ever find yourself in this same position. At least ask about it; there is no cure for lymphedema.

I hadn't been told this could happen so I did not even know what it was when it began. I wish the doctors had told me about it, but many specialists seem to know only their field, and nothing much about areas that could be affected by the work they are doing.

Everything happened so quickly that I had no time to research and prepare questions for the doctors. The Internet was barely getting started, so it would have been a lot harder then. I think one of the best things you can do is arm yourself with information and things to ask, and also alternative ways to treat it. I wouldn't advocate not using conventional western medicine. I do think of it as covering all the bases. You may even have a doctor who does know about alternative medicine.

I can't say I found a lot of humor in my situation. I did find it pretty difficult, but also much easier, after the actual operations and biopsy reports were done, to cope with than I thought it would be. I did learn to avoid the "Oh poor you" people, well-meaning as they are, as I found that kind of sympathy did me little good, except at figuring out clever ways to stay out of their paths and deflect their endless, unctuous expressions of sympathy.

And what I remember best about it all, other than the apprehension I still feel at annual mammogram time (but I would feel that way anyway), is the joy of knowing I was alive, I would be some time longer on earth, the blood singing in my veins.

Cynthia lives in State College, PA, with four cats, three of them rescues. She is not one of those crazy old ladies who will eventually acquire 150 cats. She has two great sons and is a retired Penn State teacher who loves to hang out with friends in beautiful places.

A Sprinkle of FUN from Tammy...
Martha's Way or My Way...

Martha's Way: Stuff a miniature marshmallow in the bottom of a sugar cone to prevent ice cream drips.

My Way: Just suck the ice cream out of the bottom of the cone, for Pete's sake. You are probably lying on the couch with your feet up anyway.

A Collection of Stories
Jamie Fisher

Story 1 – Angels Among Us

Melissa Knepp, the nurse navigator at the Breast Center Radiology department in Lewistown was the first angel I met during my diagnosis and subsequent journey through Breast Cancer.

It all started the day I was going for my first ultrasound. I was driving to my appointment, listening to the radio as always, when an advertisement came on about Melissa Knepp, the new nurse navigator at Lewistown Hospital Imaging Department. She was there to help people when they got the diagnosis of cancer.

At my appointment, I asked the ultrasound tech if she knew anything about the nurse navigator. She provided me with information and asked if I would like to speak to her. I was very eager because that is who I am…I want to learn everything I can about things that are going on in my world.

So the call was made and Melissa immediately came down. We talked about what was going on, what questions I had and where to go from there. Additionally she got answers for me, attended appointments with me, knew the right questions to ask the staff and guided me through the medical jargon.

Melissa got me connected with the Hershey Breast Care Center when it was determined that a double mastectomy was my best option with chemotherapy to follow.

Once I started chemo treatments and I knew I was going to lose my hair, it was Melissa who took me to our local Cancer Treatment Center and hooked me up with the perfect wig for me and different hats and scarves to wear. I was elated!

She has been with me every step of the way on my journey and we have become very close friends.

The Lord works in mysterious ways and brings people into our lives when we need them. Melissa is and always will be one of my angels.

Story 2 - God's Plan For Me

I have always been told and always believed God has a plan for each and everyone of us. Some of us go through life never knowing what that plan is. I was one of them until recently.

I had never been one of those people who felt I had to go to church to have my beliefs in God be verified. I felt as long as I had my beliefs that's all that mattered. And to a point I still feel that way.

As a child, my Mother saw to it that I went to church but there wasn't a real strong Father figure in my life to help encourage that. Don't get me wrong, my Father was there in the house while I was growing up but we didn't have much of a relationship. What can I say, it was the 60's and 70's! So when I grew older the need to go to church every Sunday wasn't there, even as I began raising my babies. My first son, Joshua, was baptized but my other three children have not been. I did take my children to church…sporadically.

I believed in God and the Father, Son and Holy Spirit, I just hadn't had the feeling that I needed to attend church every Sunday to prove it. Additionally, I hadn't found a church that I felt comfortable in and didn't feel I was being judged by the congregation.

My first recollection of questioning why God did horrible things to good people was when my Pappy got cancer when I was 11 years old. I remember lying on the couch crying and thinking "God, why did you have to take my Pappy?" I loved my Pappy very much and even though it's been almost 40 years, I miss him as much as I did when I was 11. He was a very positive influence in my life.

My next struggle with trying to understand God was when I was almost 30 with my second child Kaitlyn Taylor, a beautiful dark haired little porcelain cherub. It wouldn't be until many months later that I would learn that my precious baby girl would face a lifetime of physical obstacles. It would take 2 ½ years to find out my daughter was born with Spinal Muscular Atrophy. I was devastated…at first. I remember thinking "Why God would you do this to such a precious little child? Little did I know, he knew what his plan was for me and my beautiful daughter. He then went on to bless me with two more perfect children.

I remember talking with my best friend Patty, who passed away a couple of years ago from breast cancer (ironically) and I miss her very much also…asking God again why he would do this to me. I must have been feeling sorry for myself out of the frustrations going on in my life. Patty said "I believe God doesn't give us anymore than we can handle."

It was at that point I began thinking about her statement and ultimately came to realize my friend was right because God has thrown me many struggles and I have come out stronger with each one. But I still wasn't ready to be in his house and worshipping him regularly. I also don't think I was ready to have God fully and completely in my heart. Maybe I was still mad at him for taking my Pappy from me.

It would be many years until I would come to learn why God left a perfectly innocent little angel with the inability to run and play like all the other children. I learned to advocate for my daughter from the time she was a baby. I never treated Kate (as we call her now) any differently than my other three children. She had chores to do just like the others. And when she did something she knew she wasn't supposed to or she acted up, she got punished just like the other three. I remember one day pulling her out of her wheelchair when she was about 5 and spanking her for her behavior at the time….and my son (14 years old) looked at me and said "How can you do that to her?" I replied "her condition doesn't change anything if she misbehaves and needs a spanking, she's going to get it just like the rest of you." I'm sure Kate can attest to the fact that even when she was fighting with me about walking in her braces and walker, I was there pushing her all the way, telling her "can't" isn't in our vocabulary!

She is now an amazing, beautiful, young independent woman who has just completed her freshman year of College at Edinboro University majoring in Psychology. She wants to be a rehab psychologist in a children's hospital…giving back what was given to her when she spent long periods of time in the rehab unit following her many surgeries.

She has been a wonderful role model to kids and adults – both able bodied and not. She has told me how I am her hero (even wrote a poem about it and had it published when she was in the 6th grade), but truly she is and always will be MY hero. She is a true inspiration to anyone she meets. I am truly blessed and proud to call her my daughter. The truest example of God's plan.

The summer of 2010 proved to be my next encounter with God's Plan. I suffered from severe depression for many years. It didn't hit too much in winter but would affect me terribly in the summer. I think because summer was always special to me growing up. Every summer we would pack up and "go on vacation." Whether it was camping or going to my late Aunt Judy's in Delaware and going to be beach…we got away. We didn't have much money but we always went on vacation, and I wanted to do the same for my kids growing up. I've been a single parent for the last 10 years and I don't have to tell you how difficult saving money for anything extra can be. Most of the time I was a self-employed painter, which meant if I didn't work, I didn't get paid. …….

Story 3 - Hershey Isn't Just For Chocolate Lovers

If you mentioned the word "Hershey" to me a year ago, I would've thought chocolate. Today I think it's a city of angels. I was diagnosed with breast cancer last October during a routine mammogram. Timing was not great of course, because I had just overcome a serious depression. I see now God's hands were on my shoulders when he saved me from myself because he had a much bigger picture in mind. A beautiful picture that now encompasses a "Relay For Life" team of over 100 people. Four beautiful children (one in a wheelchair since birth) and I'm soon to be adopting a teenager with Spiral Muscular Atrophy. I have never felt stronger or better.

Don't get me wrong; this road was not an easy one. One of the biggest frustrations was playing the waiting game. When I was diagnosed, the subsequent test results seemed to take forever. A local doctor told me he thought all I needed was radiation but I had to wait for more results. In my frustration…I sought a second opinion at Hershey Medical Center and I am so grateful I did. What they told me was a whole different story. Through the help of a nurse navigator, it was recommended I have a double mastectomy. Upon hearing the news, I figured I had two choices. I could either feel sorry for my children and myself or keep a positive attitude and accept help. But keeping a positive attitude and accepting help were not easy. There were days I admitted that chemotherapy was "kicking my butt" and all I could do was cry. But I needed to cry. I also needed my caramel sundae's and hot tub soaks.

When people embark on a journey they often take pictures so I figured I might as well too. I took pictures of the wonderful people I met at every appointment and all the friends and family that cheered me on. I took my pink boa to my treatments and friends brought their pom poms. When I heard the news of a double mastectomy I told myself my breasts had served their purpose after all (I breast fed all my children). I had breast reconstruction done at the same and you can barely see my scars 6 months later. Lose my hair? Think of all the money I saved on hair color! My daughter's baseball team raised money for my Relay For Life team (Jane's Angels) by having a "Shave Your Head" party. If you would've told me a half a year ago I'd have teenage girls become my hero's I may not have believed you.

In the old days, 'cocktail hour' meant drinks with umbrellas. After surgery, 'cocktail hour' meant nausea and allergic reactions. In an effort to combat nausea, the medical team included a steroid that meant I was "wired." I had so much extra energy that after my appointments at Hershey Medical Center, I had to stop at the Hershey stores and go shopping! After my third chemotherapy "red cocktail" treatment, I shopped until 2 a.m. It was a good thing for my body and my pocketbook that they fine-tuned the combination.

In some ways, this was the worst experience and in others, the best experience. The nurse navigator and team at Hershey are true angels. I now have a photo album full of new friends and precious memories. I count every day as a blessing and realize the importance of humor. I also know I could not have made it alone, and I thank God and my "heroes" for the most incredible journey of my life.

Jamie Fisher
As written by Kathy Salloum

Jamie lives in Lewistown, PA with two children, two dogs and a cat!

A Sprinkle of FUN from Tammy...

"A male gynecologist is like an auto mechanic who never owned a car."   -- Carrie Snow

The Feather
Lori Fisher

After going through my Breast Cancer journey, I wrote this poem
in Honor of every special person who walked the path of my
journey with me. At times, carrying me.

This <u>Feather</u>
I had always thought-
now I know it to be true;
It came to me one day we were together,
as I was following you.

I saw it as it floated down,
sparkling in the sun;
And as I reached out to catch it,
I realized what God had done.

You see, God sends His angels down,
to each of us - one is meant;
I just hadn't realized it yet,
so a reminder He had sent.

This feather I return to you-
you never knew you lost it;
From your wing it gently fell,
and in my hand I caught it.

I felt the brush of your soft wing,
it was then that I knew;
When God sent my angel down-
He sent me you.

Lori makes her home in Thompsontown, PA, with her husband
Fred and son Joshua. She can be reached at
loriisawesome@hotmail.com.

The Presence of a Friend
Lisa Fritz

Friends come and go in our busy lives and many times we do not make the effort to stay in touch. In this day and age with cell phones, emails, texting and tweeting, there should not be any excuse but we always find one.

When my best friend from high school, Suzanne, and I left for college, we vowed to keep in touch. We were both going to Philadelphia and our colleges were only about 10 blocks apart. How silly now to think that we just lost touch! Looking back on that time, I guess we both got wrapped up in studies and the usual college events. Life went on and after college she married and moved out of the state. I stayed and went to medical school, residency and finally married and in practice. Out of the blue, during my residency, I received an invitation to a baby shower for Suzanne. After many years we did connect briefly at that shower. It was wonderful to see her and I was excited to hear she was having her first child. Soon after, I found out I was pregnant with my first child.

Unfortunately, as in the past, life caught up with both of us and we again lost touch. Suzanne was in Florida and I was in Pennsylvania, both with a new baby and jobs. Juggling motherhood and work took the majority of my time and despite the convenience of a new invention called "the phone", we did not keep up with our correspondence.

Surprisingly, after a few years and, for me, a few more children, Suzanne got a job and low and behold, moved to central Pennsylvania where I was living. You would think this would have fostered better communication but again life caught up with both of us and we tried occasionally to get together.

Shortly after, Suzanne remarried, I recall the phone call she made to me to tell me she had breast cancer. She was in her 30's with a young son and new husband, facing a diagnosis which frightens all women. After several surgeries and chemotherapy, we again connected. I look back now and regret I was not able to provide more support during that time. Suzanne was fiercely private and did have a network of support from her church and family. I would talk to her occasionally and even surprised her in the hospital after one of her surgeries.

Suzanne had several recurrences and during the last recurrence we did make an effort to have lunch several times. During those times I listened and heard her discuss her journey with this diagnosis. It seemed surreal and was hard to understand. I could show her support but did not truly understand the full ramification of the diagnosis and its effect on her life. When she opted to stop treatment, I actually was upset with her. Her son was entering his senior year of high school and I could not imagine "giving up." Her response to me was that her quality of life during her multiple chemotherapy sessions was not worth it for her family and for herself. She felt her son had grown up with her cancer and she was not able to try experimental chemotherapy. She wanted the last months of her life to be as "normal" as possible for her family.

I left that lunch, confused, upset and unable to grasp the entire meaning of this statement. Suzanne died three months later. Her funeral was difficult for me, especially seeing our high school yearbook open to a picture of us. It was wonderful to connect with her family. Little did I know that one year later, I, too, would have to face the demon..."breast cancer".

When I received my diagnosis in November of 2004, my first thoughts were of Suzanne and her brave fight with the disease. In fact, I recall a dream of me sitting on my couch with Suzanne next to me. I think of that dream often and know that her presence was with me during my surgeries, chemotherapy and radiation. I was able to understand her option to stop therapy as her way of keeping control of her life. When you receive the diagnosis of cancer, you are no longer in control. Your body has betrayed you. You go from one appointment to another, usually in a fog, just trying to get by and fight the disease. We are never totally in control, only God can claim that, but we as humans, do want some ability to direct our lives.

It has now been 7 years since Suzanne died and 6 years since my diagnosis. I still occasionally hear from Suzanne's mother and I think of her often. It is still surreal to think I lost a high school friend to this disease but I know during my fight and going forward, Suzanne is a silent strength for me. Maybe she is one of those angels that is there for all of us during our tough journeys. I hope someday to be that strength for others during their journey.

Through this Suzanne's inspiration, I was able to connect to several other breast cancer survivors in the area and founded a breast cancer networking group. Our mission is to support breast cancer patients from the moment they are diagnosed, through their therapies and after their treatments are completed. We have grown from a group of four women to over sixty members. We provide sunshine baskets during chemotherapy and radiation therapy and a listening ear for anyone in need. I guess you could say, Suzanne's presence during my therapies served as my "sunshine basket."

Lisa Fritz is a 6 year breast cancer survivor living in York, PA. She is co-founder of P.I.N.K. (Power in Knowledge), a local networking group for breast cancer survivors in the York area. She is married and the mother of four children.

The Wonderful Tragedy
Written by Matthew Tuckey - For My Mom
Diane Funston

A wonderful tragedy began six years ago in a single, surreal moment. As I lumbered around my college apartment, hoping, for once, to make it to a morning class on time, the ringing phone pierced the silence. I answered and heard the familiar, seemingly stressed voice of my mother on the other end.

"What are you doing?" my mother questioned. I answered quickly that I was getting ready for class, not in the mood to have an early conversation. My mother continued, "I have something to tell you…"

The next 60 seconds seemed like an eternity. My stomach dropped, my heart raced, and my head became clouded and dizzy. The room seemed to spin as I strained to listen to the monotone, rehearsed speech my mother had prepared in the language of breast cancer, lymph nodes, biopsies, and other unfamiliar terms that I could not comprehend. Just as you can recount stories from your childhood that you only remember from the telling and retelling of situations by your parents, the next words interrupted my mother's prepared lines unexpectedly, although my mind cannot recall speaking them. "Are you going to die?" I asked.

The next few chapters of this story unfolded slowly, but ultimately with a happy outcome. My mother experienced roller coaster rides of chemotherapy, radiation, struggles, tests, highs and lows. I, for the most part, stayed away. At the time, I could not deal with the reality of what was happening and of the potential consequences. I buried myself in college activities and avoided the hospital-filled home life, choosing to pray and support from afar. After waging an ongoing battle, my mother prevailed and is in her sixth year of recovery. I thank God daily that He did not take her and leave me to question why I was not there more often.

Countless similar stories such as this are played out everyday across the world. Some end triumphantly and others sadly. As I write this today, I know there are still emotions and feelings that I have not correctly or completely dealt with regarding this and other chapters in the book of my life. However, looking back on the play that is our lives, I would entitle this scene "The Wonderful Tragedy."

The tragedy is easily identified in the pain, suffering and fear that eat away at one's soul just as the cancer tries to eat away at one's body. But where can the "Wonderful" be found? Looking closely, I can brush away the dust of negativity and struggle and see a wonderful picture below.

I see a mother who has begged, pleaded, promised, questioned, sought after, and cried to God developing intimate conversation with the Creator that we should all be striving to accomplish.

I see a mother who has a distinctively new approach to her marriage, her career, her family, her friends, and her future. And, I see a son who recognizes the brevity of life and the crucial importance of making the most of every day. Anger, jealousy, and those people who irritate you like nails on a chalkboard are all situations we choose to place ourselves in. How are you going to respond, feel, react, proceed, look back or relate? You choose. No one else makes you feel a certain way. You choose. This "Wonderful Tragedy" has made me choose to strive everyday to be as brave, positive, appreciative, thankful, courageous, forgiving and optimistic as the heroine in this story.

Diane Funston
As written by Matthew Tuckey (son)

Let's Go Team
Anita "Folly" Gerstle

I have had a benign cyst, a stereotactic marker, a needle biopsy and a surgical biopsy…2008 was a roller coaster year for me. My first two grandchildren were born and I had a hysterectomy/bladder sling (in April) due to a prolapsed uterus and there were some "suspicious cells" on my mammogram.

I went through the agonizing fear imagining the worst and the shock of "Where did this come from? Cancer runs in my husband's family, heart disease runs in mine!" and "Why me?"

Then my athletic "competitive spirit" kicked in and I told myself I was going to attack whatever I had with every fiber of my being. With God's help, I will get through this.

I was one of the lucky ones, this cancer was DCIS and sort of contained in the ducts, was Stage 0 and we found it early. My husband said he would support my decisions.

In August, the surgeon removed a 1"x 2" chunk with a wide, clean margin and believes we got it all. I did not have chemotherapy or radiation but was put on Tamoxifen for 5 years.

One year after I had my surgery, I was at my family doctors for just an annual check-up and ran into a friend of mine. We chatted and caught up on news of our kids. Later I was having some routine blood work done and my friend came in and seemed agitated. I asked her, "What's wrong?" She broke down and told me she had a suspicious area in her mammogram and was paralyzed with fear. I was able to hug and comfort her with some positive encouragement that up until a year before I wouldn't have known what to say to her. It was a blessing to be at that place at that time.

And now, one of my cousins also has breast cancer, so I guess it is in my family. I have read Tammy Miller's book, *The Lighter Side of Breast Cancer Recovery* and I recommend it to anyone and everyone who is dealing with or knows someone with breast cancer.

I am a Caring Clown and I know the value of using humor to help healing. In Head First – The Biology of Hope and the Healing Power of the Human Spirit by Norman Cousins, he tells us that healing might depend on the difference between two physicians giving a diagnosis. One doctor may be brutally honest and the patient feels defeated while the other doctor can be tactfully honest and offer hope and positive encouragement. Sometimes the only difference between two cancer patients is that the one who laughs releases more T-cells that boost the immune system. And in HUMOR-The Lighter Path to Resilience and Health by Paul McGhee, PhD, he emphasized exactly what Hospital/Caring Clowns believe and the reason they do what they do: Humor helps heal!

2011 Buckle up – it's going to be a bumpy ride! In April I went to my OB-GYN for an annual check-up. He discovers a lump in an area that had been previously biopsied. (Good thing I am flat-chested – the lump showed up sooner!). His office calls the Breast Center to have a diagnostic mammogram done as soon as possible. They also did an ultrasound because of its suspicious location. I have scar tissue and tough fibers in the "remains" so it was hard to get a clear image. I wake the next day with a tension headache. My OB-GYN calls to tell me the results and then his office calls the surgeon to see if she could fit me in. I have an appointment the next day. God is so good to give me doctors who really care about me!!! I don't want to put anything off – the longer I wait to find out the results, the longer stress and tension can build. I am a "get-it-done" kind of person. I may not like the answer, but at least then I know what I'm going to have to deal with and can plan my attack.

I have the surgical biopsy done and am told, "this looks different" than before. I get results a week later. It is "more of the same" (DCIS). The recommendation is a mastectomy…I asked, "What about removing both as a preventative measure. No offense, I like you and all, but if this is going to keep coming back every few years, let's get ahead of the game." (I mentioned that I am a

Caring Clown – I gave my surgeon a red nose on my way out – she wore it back to the registration desk – her staff loved it!!!).

I went home and did some investigation on-line at the National Institutes of Health and the American Cancer Society so I was informed before I went to see the plastic surgeon for the possibility of reconstruction. After getting all of the information, I went home and made a list. I am a visual person so instead of having all the advantages and disadvantages swimming around in my head, I put them down on 3"x5" cards so I could see them. It helped me come to my decision. This is one decision that each woman will have to make for herself. It is what she decides that she wants to live with…In this case it IS all about ME! Now that the decision is made – Let's DO this and get it done! The sooner we start, the sooner we can get on with recovery, healing and the rest-of-my-life's journey!

"The wise physician doesn't minimize the seriousness of the illness; they present it as a challenge that calls for the best both doctor and patient have to offer."
LET'S GO TEAM!!!

Peace to you today and always… Anita Gerstle

Anita lives in Kettering, Ohio, with her husband Joe. They have four grown children and four grandchildren. She is a volunteer Hospital Clown at Dayton Children's Medical Center and a member of Anything But Serious Clown Troupe at Kettering Medical Center. You can reach her at jagerstle@aol.com.

Thoughts of a Breast Cancer Survivor Going Through Radiation Therapy
Madeline Goldman

Day 23 out of 35
23 times I have assumed this horizontal position. Arms above my head, Right holding left.

12 more times to walk into this room. Down the narrow hall.

2 and ½ weeks of facing this table. Making conversation with the technicians. Trying to ignore my naked chest. One breast, and one breast cut in half.

3 more meetings with the radiation oncologist.

12 more check-ins with the front desk. My name is entered into the computer. Everyone knows I am here now.

Minutes to wait until my name is called. Escorted into the room. Down the narrow hallway. Around the corner. I place my purse on the chair. Take my glasses off. Shirt and undershirt off. Everything goes on the chair.

Early on in the treatments, I chose not to change into a hospital gown before therapy. I did not want to feel as if I was a patient. I did not want to associate with the other patients. I did not want to walk past the other patient's families. I did not want to sit with the other patients in hospital gowns.

5 steps to the table. I don't bother with the towel to cover my chest any more. They have all seen my breasts. One full breast. One half of one breast. An A cup and barely an A cup.

Sharpie marks cover my chest. 3 x's and one big circle

I lay down. Arms go up. Move down a little please. I am going to move you slightly.

Don't help me. Thank you.

I see my reflection in the round machine about my head. 2 red beams are being aligned to my chest. Sharpie marks are lined up. 3 x's in turquoise blue. 1 large black circle. A very large circle. My right breast has an uncanny resemblance to the dog from Spanky and Our Gang.

Left breast covered. Right breast exposed.

Here we go. Everyone leaves the room. Lights are dimmed. Music is on.

It's just me now. I am on camera. 2 cameras. Just in case.
The machine above my head is positioned to my left.
The entrance to this room is locked. Shut. Click.

Silence. Computer screens to my right and left in my peripheral vision. Blinking out my information. Numbers. Alignments, a formula for my individual treatment. Specific notes on my arc position. I don't turn my head. Lay perfectly still. Breathe normally. This silence is broken with a buzz. The centers of the computer screens are red. A red light in my right peripheral vision.

20 seconds of buzz. I close my eyes. Breathe normally.

23 treatments have burned my skin. The blisters are in various stages of existence.
Opened, closed, weeping or scabbed. They all itch. Some are bleeding.
Are you putting the Aloe gel on?
Yes.
Are you using the Biafine cream?

Yes.
Don't scratch. I know it's itchy Ms. Goldman, but don't scratch.
You're kidding, right?
I am itchy beyond description.
All I do is scratch.

Silence.

The machine to my left rotates above and over me. It stops directly over my chest before it turns. Sound like a combination lock then continues to rotate to my right. My right breast is the destination reached.

Silence. Click. Buzz. 30 seconds of buzz. Eyes closed. Breathe normally. I'm on camera.

Silence.
The machine turns slightly. Sound like a combination lock. Stops.
Silence. Last Buzz. 20 seconds. Breathe normally. Silence.
My arms relax. I cover my right breast.

Click. The door unlocks and the technician comes to get me.
Thank you. See you tomorrow.
It's bumper to bumper.
The room, buzz, red beam, table, hallway, silence, and machine are behind me.

And in front of me.
23 in back. 12 in front.

Hope it works.

Madeline is a 6 year breast cancer survivor, diagnosed with stage 1 breast cancer in 2005. She received 35 radiation treatments. She believes she could not have survived without support from her family and friends.

My Story
Judy Greig

My name is Judy, and I am a sixty-five year old breast cancer survivor. Despite the fact that I had no previous family history of the disease and few risk factors, my cancer was diagnosed in September of 2005, by way of my annual mammogram and a stereotactic biopsy. I never felt my actual tumor. It was small and located toward the back of my chest wall. I did, however, feel that something strange was happening in my breast. I could feel occasional pins and needles sensations. Those telltale suspicions led me to get my mammogram.

My initial reaction after learning of my cancer was, "What do I do now?". At the time, my pregnant daughter lived with me. She was due to deliver a baby boy in November of 2005, and was very upset at the thought of my not being around to see my future grandson grow up.

My physician connected me to a surgeon who examined me and recommended a mastectomy. "But how could this be with only stage one cancer?", I thought. Naturally, I wanted a second opinion, which, I prayed, would tell me that I was a candidate for a lumpectory instead. My breasts were small, and the thought of losing one was grievous.

Just to reinforce the fact that God does work in mysterious ways, I ran into the grocery store on the way home from the surgeon's office and right into my good friend and mammogram technician herself. She became my angel on this journey and sent me to a second opinion service at a nearby hospital. There I met a wonderful array of expert, caring providers who answered all of my questions and helped me take charge of my disease. Being a librarian by trade, I also thoroughly researched everything I could find relating to ductal carcinoma and my personal situation.

My mastectomy took place on November 11, 2005, with my breast implant being inserted during the same surgery. Further reconstruction procedures followed over the next six months. And,

I am happy to say that I was able to attend the birth of my grandson on November 16, 2005. Now that's a quick recovery!

Throughout the entire cancer process from diagnosis to treatment I stayed strong and took charge of what was happening to my body. Since I had no spouse or partner, the decision making rested on my shoulders alone. My physicians were honest and helpful, and I never second guessed their explanations or advice. Also, my daughter accompanied me to my physician visits to make sure I was hearing all that was said. With expert help I have remained cancer free since my surgery and am now off all medications. I am a survivor and proud of it!

If my story has touched a nerve in any person reading it, may I make two strong recommendations about dealing with breast cancer. First, get those mammograms annually for early detection. And second, don't settle on treatments until you find a team of doctors in whom you have complete faith and confidence. Remain calm, trust your instincts, and put your faith in God that his will be done.

Judy is happily retired and living with her partner in Lehighton, PA. A former school librarian, she now fills her days with music (ukulele and piano), gardening, reading and dancing. She counsels other breast cancer patients through her work with Support of Survivors at Lehigh Valley Hospital.

Hair We Go
Jade Gritzfeld

Everyone has a best feature – something that people remember about us. It is the one thing that makes us smile when we look in the mirror. It may be our dimples, our eyes or our smile. My trademark feature was thick, long brown hair that flowed around me as I danced. I would tilt my head and brush it back with the flick of my wrist. Yes, anyone who knew me as an adult knew me with long hair.

From the day I was diagnosed with breast cancer up to the moment when I was wheeled into the operating room, I refused to consider chemo therapy plus hair loss. I was blindly determined to think simple: surgery, radiation, back at work in a month.

As I drifted into consciousness in the recovery room, a nurse was hanging a new IV bag. The blood pressure machine was doing a steady beep, beep – a good sign. When she emptied the drainage tubes sewn into my chest, I noticed her perfectly coiffed hair – slightly curly, nice bangs with a hint of grey mixed in the light brown colour.

"You have beautiful hair," I mumbled. She smiled. I think I smiled back as I drifted off.

"Modified radical." Those words jolted me into back into consciousness as the recovery room nurse gave report to the ward nurse. I was coherent enough to start processing the implications. Modified radical meant cancer in the lymph nodes. Chemo therapy was now in the picture. Somehow in the whirling thoughts flowing through my mind, my hair became "La Mane." Chemo therapy would cause me to lose my best feature, La Mane. I pushed the future reality out of my mind, happy with the present reality of La Mane resting on my shoulders.

A few weeks later during my first visit to the Cancer Centre, the medical oncologist reviewed chemo treatment options with me. Afterwards, his nurse said:

"Jade, let's go for a quick tour of the Cancer Centre."

"Not now," I replied. "I have a meeting. Can we please do the tour another time?" Avoidance was crucial because it would delay the inevitable.

"It won't take long." Let's go."

We headed downstairs into a reception area dominated by a large yellow and brown sign above the nursing station: CAUTION RADIATION. The people waiting were all grey-haired, wrinkled and slow-moving.

"This is where you'll go for radiation after you're done chemo."

We headed back up a different set of stairs. Each step I took was progressively slower, delaying the viewing as much as possible. With a deep breath, I walked into the chemo area to see a long row of twenty lounging-chair stations. There were real people sitting in those chairs. Some were reading. Some were sleeping. Others were visiting. Everyone wore hats or wigs except for one woman. Her scalp was half bald and half sparse hair. What remained was in splotchy clumps of different lengths. Is that how I was going to look? The future reality of losing La Mane rushed at me with an "I-can't-ignore-it-anymore" thud.

NO!!! I reached up to defiantly flick my hair back. No! If losing my hair was an eventuality, I would choose when and how it was coming off – not my disease choosing it for me. That night, I began a series of letters to La Mane. Choice is empowering. I was taking back control and separating from La Mane on my own terms. I would find the good in the bad.

Every day, I choose to look for something to celebrate. When it comes to my hair, I salute my hair stylist hero, Anita. She made arrangements for us to go to the "by appointment only" wig shop. We walked in with a goal to laugh and have fun. After all, if I knew that I would be wearing a wig and everyone else knew that I would be wearing a wig. I would shout out, "I'M WEARING A WIG!"

The first wig that I selected was "Auburn Tousled" The wig couldn't replace La Mane but men liked Auburn Tousled. To receive an ego boost on chemo therapy was a good thing. For my second wig, I chose the most deliberate red I could find, paprika. This wig was set in a nice blunt bob cut. Therefore it became Paprika Bob.

During the weeks after surgery, my friend Don and I enjoyed pleasant conversation while driving out of town. At one point, he got very serious and said, "Jade I have to tell you something that's been bothering me but I don't want to hurt your feelings." I had no idea where his statement was going.

He took a deep breath and blurted out, "I hate Paprika Bob."

OK. Men liked Auburn Tousled but didn't like Paprika Bob. I could live with that.

Armed with Auburn Tousled and Paprika Bob, my newest accessories, I wondered, "Am I ready?" When eight friends shaved their heads to raise $5,000 for cancer research, I discovered that perhaps I could find the good in the bad. I also realized that I was ready.

On the evening after my first chemo treatment, I brought my favourite bottle of red wine – a baco noir – and two crystal wine glasses to Anita's salon. It was odd going there when no one else was around. The smells were missing. The buzz of conversation was absent. Chairs were empty, except for one. Anita was waiting for me. I languished brushing La Mane one last time; starting at the top and pulling the brush down and away, feeling the flow of hair escape the brush. We opened the wine. In good Toastmaster form, I gave a toast: To my soon-to-be fallen hair.

After clinking glasses, Anita put hers down and picked up the shaver. In a gesture to soften the pending extreme change, she offered, "I can start with shaving half your head if you'd like."

"That's OK. Just do it all."

Anita started at the widows peak in the centre of my forehead, pulling along my scalp all the way down to my neck. I could still feel the hair on my back but it was no longer attached. Strip by strip, the hair dropped. By the time Anita was done, La Mane carpeted the floor.

Being newly bald was a curiosity for me. Anita kept commenting on the nice shape of my head. She said that my mom turned me well. I had no idea what that meant. Later as more moms and grandmas made the same comment, I learned that when mothers turn their babies while they sleep, it helps create a nicely shaped head.

We stared at the bald head in the mirror, Anita's hands resting on my shoulder. I looked at her and saw tears brimming in her eyes. I smiled and touched her hand. I had made peace.

I didn't need my hair. It would grow back. Instead, I celebrated a special moment with my hair stylist hero. We sipped more wine, trying on Auburn Tousled and Paprika Bob. Then, with Paprika Bob covering my head, I walked out the door, celebrating and relishing life because I did find the good in the bad.

Jade Gritzfeld is a speaker and trainer dedicated to making her community a better place. She spends her time helping small businesses and teaching entrepreneurs. You can contact her through www.gritzfeld.com.

A Sprinkle of FUN from Tammy...

A woman never forgets her age once she decides what it is.
-- Unknown (but it could be from any of us – including Jade ☺ !!)

My Story
Katherine M. Gross

In July of 1996, at age 39, I had an appointment with my GYN to have a lump I found under my armpit checked out. Prior to this, in November 1995, I had just had my yearly mammogram and was given a "thumbs up" - nothing was found. After going through six weeks of antibiotics, thinking I had an infection due to the "aluminum" in my deodorant, it was determined that there was something more serious going on. With a biopsy, the diagnosis was found to be early stage II breast cancer - that had spread to 10 out of 10 lymph nodes tested. A radical mastectomy was performed on the right side followed by intense chemotherapy and radiation.

Some when they hear the word cancer think DEATH and others think LIVE. I thought death at first, but I felt in my heart that God had more for me to do…what, I didn't know exactly.

Six years later, in May 2002, a mammogram detected a suspicious spot on my left side. It was determined to be stage II breast cancer, a different type than the first. In July, I had another radical mastectomy and had to once again go through chemotherapy and radiation.

I can't tell my story without telling you of God's blessings in my life and giving Him the credit for all that He has done for me! I thank God for my faith and belief in Him that has sustained me this far. As a Believer in God and His healing power, I stand on His promises found in the Word of God that "…all things work together for the good to them that love the Lord and are called according to His purpose." (Romans 8:28)

I believe there is a reason for everything that happens to us in our life. We may not understand the reasoning right away, but I believe that "we will understand it better by and by". There is a reason for my being where I am today.

One of my mottos is – "if you are given a lemon, make lemonade". In good or not so good health, everyday is a blessing from God, so LIVE every minute to the fullest. I look at each path my life takes as a new chapter in "Kathy's Book of Life" and an opportunity to be used by God to either help someone else or to make a change for good in this world. I've learned not to "sweat the small stuff," but to deal with what I can change and pray for God's help and guidance in the things I can't.

In the African-American community, I often hear, "what I don't know won't hurt me". But the sad fact is breast cancer can kill if not detected early. While black women are less likely to develop breast cancer, we have the highest age-adjusted mortality rates from breast cancer of any racial/ethnic group in the United States. One of the main reasons for this mortality disparity, experts say, is that Black women are diagnosed at more advanced stages of the disease. In other words, we wait too long.

Ladies, our body…our temple, belongs to God, let's protect it…get your mammogram!

Kathy lives in Harrisburg, PA and has been married to Jonathan, Sr. for 37 years. They have three grown children, seven grandchildren and one great grandchild. Kathy is employed by the Commonwealth of PA.

A Sprinkle of FUN from Tammy…

"The hardest years in life are those between ten and seventy."
-- Helen Hayes (at 73)

Dancing to Health
Honi Gruenberg

Once I began a family of my own, I ignored my health for many years. I was always so busy with my kids and work that I never took the time to ensure my own well-being. Because I hadn't gone for a mammogram in so long, in 1998, a friend of mine urged me to schedule one. I had every intention of doing so, but ultimately had to cancel for a business trip. During that travel, I felt a lump and realized it was growing. Upon my return, it was discovered that the lump was, in fact, breast cancer. Initially, I was very angry with myself for not prioritizing my health. I felt that I should have paid more attention to all of the signs. To help me feel more empowered, I have since become involved in various organizations; I regularly attend events such as Race for the Cure and Relay for Life and I began a support group. Being involved in these activities makes you realize how truly strong you are, and how courageous other women can be. It is an amazing bonding experience.

The women in the support group have all been wonderful. It is inspiring to listen to stories about how far they have come, and how much they appreciate life. I have spent time with women just before they succumbed to the disease and to have that sisterhood is truly remarkable. I also met my best friend, Mary Jo, at the support group, who was one of my biggest sources of motivation. She was a few months ahead of me in the process, so she was able to talk me through a lot of things – she let me know when I could start coloring my hair again!

I also began learning to belly dance. There was a program called "Focus on Healing" which utilized dance moves to help the lymphatic system. I have studied this program for 6 years, although I still want to stand in the background! (I've been told that I make use of my facial muscles more than my stomach!) That experience has been so much fun, and I never would have taken part in it, had it not been for breast cancer.

A funny memory that always gives me a laugh is thinking about one day right after I had reconstruction for my mastectomy. Things didn't quite "match up," and I caught myself walking around my house singing, "One of these things is not like the other…" from Sesame Street. Cancer is obviously a serious disease, but you have to learn that you can't take yourself so seriously.

Honi Gruenberg
As written by Kelsey Itak

Honi's second life started in 1998 when she was diagnosed with breast cancer. She became involved with wonderful organizations such as the Pennsylvania Breast Cancer Coalition, American Cancer Society, Rotary, Pink Light Walk and Congregation B'nai Harim. While working at Oracle Corporation, she has found that there is enough time in the day to give back to the many people who come in touch with this disease. It is their strength, wisdom, courage and humor that drives her. Honi is extremely proud of her children David and his wife Christina and daughter Elizabeth and her husband Chris. She is blessed with wonderful family and friends and lives in Effort, PA with her very significant other, Robert Spady.

Checkerboard Hair
Deb Haggerty

The evening of the day my hair started to fall out, Christie, Barbara and I were having dinner at one of our favorite restaurants. Naturally, I had to tell them how it all happened.

"Guess what happened this morning?"

"What happened, Deb?" Christie asked, leaning forward in anticipation.

"I reached up to pull some fuzz out of my hair and the whole clump of hair came out. I'm losing my hair!"

"Wow! What did you do?"

"I kept pulling pieces from different places on my head – then I showered and washed my hair to see how much more would come out."

Christie was fascinated. Barbara was unnaturally quiet.

"You know what would be fun?" I said, "Let's go back to my house after dinner, sit on the deck, and see if we can make a checkerboard pattern on my head!"

"How can you talk like that!!?" Barbara shouted at us. Our heads whipped around as we looked at her with astonishment. "She's losing her hair! That's terrible!" Barbara was near tears.

"It's her hair, Barbara," Christie murmured soothingly. But Barbara was not to be comforted. She had too many friends who had cancer – the reminder that I was another was the last straw.

I didn't realize right away that many people would be distraught about losing their hair. I had to learn about it from others. Hair loss seemed to be the final straw – we lose our breast(s), our energy, our stamina – why our hair, too?

When I spoke at a conference not long ago about my experiences, for example, one of the women from the audience told me how it was for her. She just shook her head, "I couldn't bear to lose my hair – it's who I am – my whole image of me is wrapped up in how I look with my hair!" Her hair was her identity – losing it meant losing herself to the disease.

I was lucky that way. My image isn't tied to the way my hair looks. In fact, one of my favorite pictures of me from that time shows me bald, with a full set of braces, and glasses instead of contacts (chemo interfered with my contacts). For me, one of the hardest adjustments was not being able to do all the things I was used to doing.

I hated the "nap attacks" and not being able to just get up and go do the things I love to do. I found that my identity was tied up in being a doer. Not doing was hard and having to ask for help was harder, much harder for me than worrying about how my hair looks.

Even so, losing my hair meant something else that many of us with cancer have to deal with. Until we lose our hair, most of us look fairly normal. Losing our hair is the step that firmly sets us apart from the rest of the population. Of course, I always had fun with it. I walked into a hair salon with a friend one day and told the shocked people that I was there for a permanent!

We'll always be apart from non-cancer folks. Once you've had breast cancer, even if you're free of symptoms for years, you know that it can always recur. As a friend said to me, "Once you've had breast cancer you can't be sure it won't come back until you die of something else."

That's the shadow that's always lurking around the corner. It's also the reality that puts other things, like being bothered by asking for help, or losing your hair, into perspective.

For me the hair issue was easily solved. A few days after that dinner with Christie and Barbara, I decided to shave my head. First, I went to the beauty parlor and got "buzzed." Then I went home and borrowed my husband's shaving cream and razor and shaved the stubble off to be truly "bald." When it started to grow back in, as I was still on chemo, I shaved it again – amazing how many different directions hair grows!

I didn't stay bald, but I did find that I liked short hair. Everyone who gets breast cancer has lots of hard things they have to deal with. But for me, checkerboard hair was one of the easy ones.

Deb's Writing...
Music Of The Tube

It was early February, 2000, and while everybody else was getting ready for Valentine's Day, I was getting ready for a full battery of tests, including my first MRI. I was in a bit of a funk.

Earlier in the week, I got the reports from a pelvic ultrasound my doctor had recommended. The "lesions" he'd seen on the CT scan I'd had recently seemed to be cysts, but he wasn't sure. One ovary was greatly enlarged by this "mass."

I had done a lot of research on the net and talked to my doctor and I knew this might be more cancer. Breast cancer and ovarian cancer often go hand in hand.

I was devastated. I had been feeling really good about making a great recovery from breast cancer surgery, but now it looked like a hysterectomy might be in my future.

I moped around the house on Tuesday night, all of Wednesday and Wednesday night thinking about maybe having a whole new kind of cancer. I didn't even get dressed. Finally I found the strength to call the doctor and schedule more tests.

Thursday I was in a much better mood. I'd taken some action and scheduled the tests for Friday. Plus, I was thinking about all my friends who were there for me and praying for me. Life might not be good, but with friends and faith it usually doesn't stay too bad for too long.

By now I was used to tests so I wasn't nervous about most of them. They started Friday morning at 7:30, way before I usually even get up. The first test was the MRI. The prospect made me nervous.

I'm just a little bit claustrophobic, and the idea of being stuck inside a really small space was scary. But the staff did everything they could to make me comfortable.

They covered me with a blanket for warmth and gave me ear plugs for the noise they said I would hear. Then they gently pushed me into a narrow tube. The quick look I took showed about 5-6 inches of space between my face and the tube.

I kept my eyes shut most of the time!! One time though, I opened my eyes and found that it was light inside the tube, at least above my face. That helped. Don't ask me why, but I didn't really feel closed in.

Then the MRI started: Tap, tap, tap - like a drummer counting cadence on the rim of a snare drum. Then loud discordant sounds: sort of a doo-wop, doo-wop, doo-wop coupled with a low pitched busy signal.

This went on for what seemed like about 10 minutes. Slight pause, tap, tap, tap and different pitches of static like you get on a TV station after it goes off the air. I kept myself amused trying to imagine what tones would be next.

Then I was wheeled out, given a dye injection, and wheeled back in for "three more sets!" By then I was used to it, and listened to the "music" - I even got to see some of the pictures. They looked pretty to me, but I would have to wait until the following week for results.

So I set off for the rest of the day's tests, with one more thing I could check off life's list. I had had my first MRI and survived by listening to the strange "music of the tube."

Deb lives in Plymouth, MA, with her husband, Roy; mom, Shirley Ogle (also a breast cancer survivor); and Coki and Foxy the Dogs. You can reach her at www.PositiveHope.com, her website designed to encourage women with breast cancer who want to control their own healthcare and family and friends who want to accompany them on their journeys.

A Pink Ribbon Story
Carole Hall

It was May 2004. As I was bathing, I noticed that something did not feel right. Was it a lump? An appointment with my gynecologist necessitated a mammogram. It was, however, several weeks between the time my doctor felt the lump and the time the mammogram was done. The waiting was not easy. I waited only to be confirmed that the news was real – I had breast cancer.

I have never been married. I have no children. Although I was always closer to my Mom, I remember my Dad holding my hand and saying "we'll get through it together". Over the next few months I was feeling like I was just getting to know my Dad. Within six months of my diagnosis, however, he passed away. I got mad at him, even though he was no longer with me. He told me we would get through this together, but he let me down. I continue to wonder today if he would still be here if he hadn't had the stress of my illness.

The next several months became very difficult because everything was happening at once. My favorite Aunt had died during the same month that I had learned of my breast cancer. I was then faced with having hysterectomy surgery. I still question the necessity of this procedure as no ovarian cancer was found. I am now, however, sterile. Having had a mastectomy and being sterile, I continue to question my attractiveness to the opposite sex. Next, I was faced with a ten-day hospital stay for an obstructed bowel. This time in the hospital, I believe, was the worst of my challenges. It does not end here. During the second round of my chemotherapy, the drugs I was given caused me to go into congestive heart failure. This was a low period of my life.

My support line was small – my Dad, while he was living, my Mom, and some people from church who came out of the woodwork. My brother, and only sibling, lived in Maine and wasn't available to help. The people from my church helped my Mom and Dad with my transportation to and from the hospital.

143

My Mom was my emotional and moral support. She was always there to listen. She has now since passed too. I am now alone.

Times were tough, but I survived! I have been in remission for six years. Because I am still here, I want others to know that cancer is not a death sentence. When I attend the local breast cancer support group, I am in the company of newly diagnosed individuals as well as long-time survivors. It is those long-time survivors who give others hope.

Carole Hall
As written by Diane Weller

Carole lives in Butler, PA, with her dog, Tucker, and her cat, Black Magic. She works in the dietary department of Butler Memorial Hospital. She can be reached at cshall@zoominternet.net Check out her website at www.carolesvirtualvscrapbook.com

A Sprinkle of FUN from Tammy...

"There is no more creative force in the world than the menopausal woman with zest."   -- Margaret Mead

My Pink Ribbon Story
Patricia Hallam

1,200 words or less? Right now I am practically wordless but in a minute I will find my voice and keeping those words to 1,200 or less will be a heroic effort. A routine mammogram a few weeks ago led to further investigation of my right breast with more scans, an ultra sound and a large core biopsy. Ouch, I needed extra numbing juice and the third try was finally an ouch less procedure.

Even before my pathology reports were completed I was on the internet researching the topic of breast cancer – after all that's what the doctors were screening me for. I went to the NIH (National Institute of Health) site and looked up Clinical Trials and noted that a doctor in the Lehigh Valley was participating in one. His name, Aaron Bleznak. I ran a Google search of his credentials and decided if my diagnosis came back breast cancer he was the doctor I wanted to consult.

Well the call came in this morning April 25th 2011 and the diagnosis is "favorable" [I smile at the term as it reminds me of a weather report that says conditions are favorable for a tornado] not good news but you better prepare and take cover, for Ductal Breast Cancer. The lovely nurse from the breast center is still waiting for my meltdown which may come but right now it is an inconvenience to worry about what is already a confirmed report. I told her that I had researched a surgical oncologist who specializes in Breast Cancer and I wanted an appointment to see him. I find that for me to get all my ducks in order eases my concerns and from what I read of this doctor's approach to medicine he's the one for me. Sight unseen he evokes confidence, compassion and expertise. Someone I can trust who will tell me all I need to know and more and then trust him with my life or at least my right breast.

My research led me to Tammy's writings and website and this book in progress. My pink ribbon story is so new I have only just begun my trip but I think I've found a trusted guide in this doctor and the people whose lives have been impacted by him. I get to see him next Monday so I have 7 days to continue my research via internet. I may even get a chance to read one of Tammy's books. I wonder if I should show up for that visit in a pink boa?

My first visit with the surgeon was a winner. And I did have Tammy's book with me. He was everything I thought he'd be and more. Very patient and an excellent communicator. I discovered I am not the pink boa kind of gal, I bought one and decided to give it to my 5 year old granddaughter to wear with her pink princess costume. But I do love to make people smile and feel good so I approached the local candy maker in town and requested he make up a box of chocolate boobs as an ice breaker gift to the new doctor and his staff. Mr. Callie makes all sorts of novelty chocolates in dark, milk and white varieties. If you're ever in Mountainhome, PA be sure to stop in and visit his shop he has trays of samples, does a candy making demonstration and has baskets of "Dolly Parton" shaped lollipops. Since I wasn't looking to buy lollipops I requested a pound of just boobs and he gladly made some for me. I did however buy one lollipop attached a pink ribbon to it and presented my gift to Dr. Bleznak after my initial consultation. It was quite a hit and I'm sure I made a lasting impression.

It turned out that I was a candidate for the clinical trial which he was running at LVH and it included MRI studies with a cryoblation treatment [basically freeze the tumor to death] followed by a lumpectomy and a sentinel node biopsy. Before the lumpectomy I was rated at Stage I Invasive Ductal Cancer but after the successful surgery and node biopsy I was assigned to Stage II because the sneaky cancer cells had invaded the sentinel node. A PET Scan revealed no other node involvement so now we wait for another test to determine whether hormones only or chemo and hormones will be the next step. Meanwhile I am still distributing candy and when I went for my cryoblation every one in the room [all 8 of them] got a pink ribboned Dolly Parton pop. This is really good candy and should be eaten but I understand many recipients are saving them as some sort of souvenir.

I am past my 2 surgeries and 3 weeks into recovery. My right boobie feels better every day although gravity and bumpy roads are still an issue. One can tense up a muscle to keep it from bouncing up and down but boobie tissue just bounces. I told the doctor it feels like trying to keep a bag of jello motionless.

The journey is still new, and my story continues... Maybe more for Tammy's next book...

Patricia lives in Mountainhome, PA a lovely scenic mountain village in the Pocono Mountains of North Eastern Pennsylvania, with her husband of 45 years, Hank. They 3 grown children, 2 sons and a daughter, a son-in-law, a daughter-in-law and 3 beautiful granddaughters, Jessica 15, Brielyn 5 and Bethany 2. 2 Families live in New England, CT and NH and the bachelor lives in LA, CA. She has 1 cat and many wildlife visitors who come to share the cat's food. One night a Possum was waiting at the back door another night you could smell the skunk and one morning a large raccoon was feeding out of the cat's dish. "Pocono Beef", better known as White Tail Deer, graze in her yard and her husband calls the flowers they set out each summer deer candy. Black Bear roam in the yard as well and the game warden calls them Callie's Bears as they often get into his dumpster looking for discarded chocolate. You can call Pat at 570-595-7169 anytime to chat or read her latest updates at http://www.caringbridge.org/visit/hankhallam a website for those who face serious health issues and want to keep family and friends informed.

Moving Forward
Beth Hamilton

Like many, my story began with a small lump. I was two years behind on my mammogram when I felt the small lump in my breast. I really thought it was nothing but my husband was persistent that I needed to have it checked. It was near the holidays in 2006 and the "nothing" lump turned out to be invasive breast cancer in my left breast. It was estrogen positive, Her 2 neu positive and about 3 cm in size.

Although it was the holidays, my mind was focused on what was happening inside my body. Unfortunately, everyone else seemed to be in holiday mode and I had a very difficult time getting answers to my many questions. This delay caused great concern as I had to make some important decisions about my treatment path. I think I was even more surprised because I am a member of the medical community. As a medical technologist I know how valuable information is to the patient and I felt very frustrated that I could not get answers from anyone.

When I finally made my decisions, my doctor tried to get a clear margin to see what was going on, but after two tries, it was determined that they could not get a clear margin so I had a mastectomy. One thing that really surprised me was that I was sent home the same day as my mastectomy. I think this is a real shame and I hope to see this changed sometime soon. I don't think I was ready to go home and deal with all that was happening. The rest of my treatment path was chemotherapy, herceptin and an aromatase inhibitor. Fortunately, there was no lymph node involvement or metastasis.

Ironically, at the same time my boss, Wendy, was also going through breast cancer. Wendy wasn't of an age to be getting a regular mammogram, so by the time her cancer was diagnosed; it was a completely different situation. I had made the decision to go through chemo and my first chemo treatment was Wendy's last. She sat with me through the treatment, which meant a great deal because I was really scared, and she helped calm my anxiety.

I know everyone has different experiences. For me, the chemo wasn't absolutely awful, as I had expected. I worked the entire time I was going through treatments and the worst one was the next to last treatment.

I knew when I started receiving chemotherapy that I would almost surely lose my hair and I thought I was prepared for that. It didn't happen right away so I was sort of hoping beyond hope that maybe I would be one of the lucky ones and maybe only have it thin out a little. One morning I was in the shower washing my hair just like any morning and without warning my hair came out in my hands in large clumps. It wasn't a gradual thing like a little bit every day on my pillow, but one day it is perfectly fine and the next morning it is gone. I was in shock. I just stood there naked staring at this huge ball of hair in my hand and started screaming for my husband. He came running since he thought something had to be terribly wrong. He opened the shower door and saw me holding this "creature" in my hand and saw the horror in my eyes. He didn't say a word. He just gently took the hair that was in my hand and left. He came back right away with a plastic bag and placed it inside. As I stood there and cried he quietly and lovingly took each new clump of hair and placed them in the bag. He understood that to just throw it away would have been painful for me. I already had a wig bought for the inevitable so it wasn't that he thought I might need it. He just knew the right thing to do at the time.

The one thing this showed me is that it's important to allow your loved ones to help you through this. It not only helps you but helps them as well and your relationships can come out so much stronger than they would have if your lives had not been touched by cancer.

It seemed as though my whole life at the time was just a little "off". Just before I was diagnosed, my brother died of leukemia. On the very same day I was diagnosed, my other brother was diagnosed with prostate cancer. And, dear Wendy did not survive her breast cancer. It was a year I could certainly have done with out, but a year of lessons and learning.

For a long time I suffered from "survivors guilt". I just could not figure out why Wendy, younger than me, would not survive this terrible illness but I would. I was just plain angry! I wouldn't get involved and would not participate in anything related to breast cancer. As time went on, I realized that it wasn't a choice that I made and it was not my fault. For whatever reason, Wendy was gone and I had work to do.

Having cancer taught me to slow down in life. Before this, I would stress over deadlines and all that "had" to be done in life. After this, I realized that it was okay for some things to wait. The housework would be there tomorrow and some things that seemed to be so important before this really wasn't important at all.

I am certainly more accepting in my life now and I try to reach out to others whenever I see someone in need. I was a person who thought I could control everything, (some even called me a "control freak" – lovingly, of course) but now I realize that I can't control everything and that is okay, too.

One of my goals from this experience is to make healthcare information more accessible to people. I was surprised and frustrated that I could not get the answers that I needed and I work hard now to help others get their needed answers. I sit on a breast cancer advisory board and this experience has given me the opportunity to know from a very personal perspective that there are ways that we can make a difference in the lives of others.

It is vitally important for people to be informed on what is happening with their treatment and their body. We deserve to get a second and even third opinion, if that is what we need. Seek out the answers and do not stop until you get what you need to make the best decision possible for yourself. You have to be your own advocate.

Through the experience I have also laughed. With the sadness there were also times of humor. One way to look at this was that I was getting a boob job and my insurance was paying for it!! So, of course I opted for a little larger size!

My family was very supportive and this meant more than they could possibly know. When something like this happens, people want to help. I always tell people, "Let them"! Some many people want to do "something" and do not know what they can do. Let people help by cooking or cleaning or whatever you need. People want to feel needed and this helps them feel like a part of what is going on in your life.

I often reflect on Wendy and why she isn't here to write her story, but I know she helped people she has left behind and there is a purpose for everything that happens in life. I know I am a better person, a stronger woman, for having this experience and I am thankful for my family and friends and each new day that I can reach out and make a difference in the life of someone else.

Dedicated to Wendy Van Dyke

Beth Hamilton
As written by Tammy Miller

Beth was 48 years old when she was diagnosed. She is originally from the Pittsburgh, PA area but has lived in the Gettysburg, PA area for over 30 years. She has a wonderful, loving husband and six outstanding sons. She says that her family is a bit of "Yours, Mine and Ours".

A Sprinkle of FUN from Tammy...

"I refuse to think of them as chin hairs. I think of them as stray eyebrows."
                    -- Many sources, but one of my personal favorites

High Anxiety
Mary Ann Hazel

Back in September, 2003, I underwent a right mastectomy with latissimus dorsi reconstruction and saline implant at a large teaching hospital. This followed the second time being diagnosed with cancer (DCIS & LCIS), which followed the initial diagnosis in 2001 (radiation and lumpectomy).

The mastectomy decision was easy to make that time. I declared I wasn't going to live in fear from mammography-to-mammography. Cancer was such a wake up call. It was at 46 years old that I started to understand the value of exercise. The sunrises and sunsets became memorable. I started to appreciate people more, loved more deeply, deepened my faith practices.

The pre op process went well, my questions were answered. I took time off from my job as a staff nurse (different hospital). On the morning of the surgery, one of the residents was making small talk in the pre op holding area. His response to my question if he slept well: he said he was awake all night being on call! After some OJ, he'd be fine. The nurse anesthetist was starting my IV at this time; I asked her to "fill me up!" The surgery went as planned.

The next morning while connected to IVs, foley catheter and automatic stockings, 5 residents make *early* morning rounds and ask if I'm ready to go home. (The surgeon had assured me in the office prior to surgery that I'd be hospitalized 48 hours). The team discontinued the IV analgesic and switched me to an oral agent. A few minutes after receiving the pill, I started itching from head-to-toe.

During the course of this morning I kept hearing movie-type music in my head. In my altered state of mind, I identify it: the Mel Brooks movie "High Anxiety". I felt like I was in a swirling vortex like the cover photo shows! I knew I wasn't thinking like a nurse. The nurse that was assigned to me during day shift told me the head-to-toe itching was my anxiety! How could I survive 5 ½ hours of surgery but think I'd not survive the post op course!   The nurse urged me to ambulate in the hallway. Fortunately another nurse saw me, told me to return to my room, that she'd give me medicine for the allergic reaction!

Humor is important to me. In the years since I've found humor to be therapeutic. I gave copies of "High Anxiety" to the surgeon and two residents. It's strange receiving care versus giving care in a hospital setting.

In 2004 I had a prophylactic left mastectomy with reconstruction and saline implant at the same large teaching hospital with the same doctor, some of the residents were different. The same nurse was assigned to me post op. There have been a few complications, but no regrets about the surgeries. At this writing I'm cancer-free.

In the movie, Mel Brooks is a psychiatrist at an institute where there are "suspicious" incidents. The movie is a comical homage of famous Hitchcock scenes. There is a segment where Brooks' Dr. Thorndyke sings the title song to a jazz tune. He sings of giving into anxiety, you "win". There were times over the years when anxiety did win. With the gift of time and guidance from others comes wisdom and understanding. It was following times in the hospital that I've gained insight into the notion that *I don't have to understand everything*! Giving up control and truly allowing the thoughts and prayers of others to carry me during those low points focused energy better spent in more positive directions. Then, healing can open up avenues of being able to receive and process information, when understanding can truly occur. It is wonderful being able to appreciate Mel Brooks' gift of comedy and laughing about anxiety.

Mary Ann has been married to her (first) husband for 32 years. Currently enjoying the "empty nest", they are the parents of a daughter and son. She has been the traditional "pastor's wife" until the difficult economy rendered her husband no longer in the parish. The rough economy pushed her back into the work force after a voluntary eight year "retirement" from nursing. She leads a monthly women's cancer support group at a hospital in

Lehighton, PA. She is a member of Trinity Lutheran Church and participates in "church lady" activities. Mary Ann can be contacted via email: mann17@ptd.net.

A Sprinkle of FUN from Tammy...

"Old age ain't no place for sissies." -- Bette Davis

A Blessed Life
Eileen Herrold

It was early March 2009, and time for my yearly mammogram...no big deal. Having a family history of breast cancer (an aunt and a sister), I was very vigilant about what I considered my yearly duty to myself.

After the mammogram was completed I went back to work, fully expecting to hear that it was negative. But instead, I was informed that they wanted me to return for further views. While this made me slightly apprehensive, I wasn't terribly concerned. Because I'm a nurse, I've had to call other women with that same message. Each time I stressed that, in most cases, it's nothing. But, I've always thought that it's much easier to be the nurse than the patient.

After more views, I was informed that I would need a needle biopsy of both breasts. By now, I was concerned and a bit scared. The results were not at all what I wanted to hear. The right breast lesion was benign, but the left breast lesion was malignant.

Hearing that you have cancer certainly is devastating news. It is such a relief to have a strong faith in difficult times. After that, things happened quickly. I saw the surgeon the same day that I got the diagnosis. I was still somewhat in a state of shock, so I was very glad that my husband was along. I felt very fortunate that I was able to have my husband or sister (who has been through the breast cancer experience herself) at my side throughout my journey.

That appointment was very soon followed by two surgeries (a month apart), fifteen months of chemotherapy and targeted therapy, and seven weeks of radiation. I spent a lot of time on the couch, too weak to do much more than force myself to eat, and get a quick shower before falling into bed.

My lowest time was when I was already feeling very weak from the chemotherapy, and developed blood clots from my port. This meant that Coumadin was added to the already long list of medications that I was taking. I remember thinking that while I thought that I would be cured of the cancer, I could die from a pulmonary embolus.

What a blessing it was to know that the Lord was with me in bad times as well as good. It meant so much to receive cards, meals (when I was too weak to cook), visits, and prayers. My church even gave me a basket with gift cards to many restaurants. Since I wasn't cooking, and my appetite was lacking, it was wonderful to occasionally get up from the couch and go out to eat (when I felt able), or have my husband bring home whatever appealed at the time.

I am now two years from my diagnosis and doing well. I don't think that a person can get a diagnosis of cancer (or any other life-threatening disease) and not have it change their life. But, we all have the ability to choose how we respond to the challenge. I've chosen to be very thankful for each new day, and I try to spend it wisely.

I can't say that there was much humor early on, but there have been a few laughs since. I asked the surgeon if he could give my right breast the same youthful uplift that I got from the lumpectomy on my left breast! Sometimes, you just have to try to make the best of a bad situation. Then, there were the musings of my "ever the joker" brother-in-law. After hearing of an upcoming karaoke contest, he suggested that my sister (his wife) and I should enter under the billing of "Una (my sister, who had had a mastectomy) and Divette" (me, who had had a lumpectomy). We all got a good laugh from that one!

At the beginning of my journey, it felt as though life would never be "normal" again. And, there is now no such thing as a routine mammogram. But, with the help of the Lord, doctors, family and friends, I am doing well. This week I was blessed with my second beautiful grandchild...what greater joy?

P.S. Please get your yearly mammogram!

Eileen is married to Jeff and they have a son, daughter, granddaughter and grandson. They reside in Julian RD, PA. Eileen is an RN, but is presently not employed.

Never Ho-Hum
Sharon A. Hill

Ho hum. Year after year I faithfully got my annual mammogram. I showed up at the radiology clinic, showed my insurance card, changed into the skimpy little dressing gown (leaving the front open and tying in the back), walked into the cold room, got my boobies squished as the technician took x-rays, sat and waited for the technician to let me know that the x-rays are acceptable, got dressed and went home. Year after year, I got the report in the mail advising me that the results are always the same... "No sign of cancer." Yippeee. It's just as I expected. No surprises. I'll be back next year.

But ten years ago, I followed the same ritual, and got a different result in the mail. I froze, read the results again and again. It's a blur to me now, but the words were something like "An abnormality was found. Please return for another visit." No ho hum this time.

I couldn't breathe. I could barely stand. What does this mean? Do I have cancer? Am I going to die? I clasped the letter, slumped into a chair, and just continued to read it over and over. My dread transformed itself into numbness. I must have sat and stared at a wall for over an hour. I found myself too numb to cry. I felt like my head was filled with cotton. Nothing to do but contemplate the worse.

When my husband got home, I somberly told him the bad news. I interpreted the letter from the radiology clinic as my death knell. My husband empathized with my fear, and had the presence of mind to ask, "When are you going back for the new set of x-rays?"

Gosh. I hadn't thought of that. I was so busy feeling sorry for myself, it never occurred to me to call for the follow-up appointment. Because the clinic was closed when I got the letter, I knew I had to call the next day. All that night, I was in a blue funk. How can I sleep knowing that my body was conspiring against me?

The Big C. CANCER. How terrifying. My poor mother. How would she take this awful news? Would my husband remarry after I was gone? Were all my insurance papers in order? Should I start planning my funeral? Which dress should I wear into eternity? Would I lose all my hair? If so, should I start looking at wigs? Would I be buried with my glasses on? What music do I want to have played at my funeral? Should I choose somber songs, like "Take my Hand, Precious Lord" or make the ceremony more upbeat with songs like "I Can See Clearly Now." Ah, me. So much to do and so little time.

The next day I called the radiology clinic and made an appointment to return for a new set of x-rays. Unfortunately, I had to wait seven days because the clinic schedule was packed. Darn. I was hoping they could make an exception for me since it was obvious to me that I was knocking at death's door. The next seven days were torture for me. I found no humor in anything. Food had no taste. Even with no taste, I decided I may as well eat everything that I usually avoided. After all, what difference would it make if I gained a few pounds prior to starting chemotherapy?

For seven tortuous days, I continued to go to work at IBM. I was hoping that I could concentrate on my daily work tasks: back to back meetings; being available to my staff; providing status to my management team; going to lunch with clients; sharing breakfast and dinner with my husband; etc, etc.. Although I was going through the motions of everything being wonderful in my life, the truth was I was sleepwalking. Each sunny day morphed into a gray fog to me. I was consumed with my mortality. I guess the palm reader I met years ago was wrong when she told me I had a long lifeline; as was the astrologist who told me that she saw me growing gracefully into old age and dying in a foreign country. (She, also, warned me to be careful around water. So, I assumed I'd walk into the bright white light after drowning in a river in France or being on an ill-fated cruise ship in the Mediterranean.)

Well, I guess it wasn't meant be. My demise would not take place in some exotic, foreign country. No, based upon the letter from the radiology clinic, I'd probably end up in a hospice. I was thinking I wouldn't allow friends to be with me in my last days because I'd probably look awful.

Finally, the day came for my follow-up appointment. I slowly walked up the stairs of the radiology clinic, showed my insurance card, changed into the skimpy little dressing gown (leaving the front open and tying in the back), walked into the cold room, get my boobies squished as the technician took x-rays, sat and waited for the technician to let me know that the x-rays were acceptable, got dressed and went home. Before I left, the technician, detecting my anxiety, promised me the clinic would call me as soon as the results were analyzed rather than have me wait for a letter.

I got the phone call two days later. I listened with shaking hands as I fought tears waiting to hear the words that would control my fate. Each word came to me as if being poured from molasses." No-sign-of-cancer."

What? Was I hearing this correctly? This time I collapsed from exhaustion and shock from hearing good news. How can this be? Would I need to return for a third test to confirm this diagnosis?

After all was said and done, the good news continued to be good news. I would not have to return for another set of x-rays. The technician said that more than one doctor reviewed the x-rays and agreed that there was no sign of cancer.

In retrospect, I wondered if the deodorant I had on during the first set of x-rays had contaminated those x-rays. You can bet I make sure I have on NO deodorant when I go for mammograms these days.

Now it was time for reflection. Based upon my receiving the first letter advising me to return to the clinic for a second set of x-rays, I jumped to the illogical conclusion that I was going to die. It is okay to be nervous about something so serious, but I took it to an extreme. I think of all the time I wasted during the seven day waiting period seeing only the dark side of life. More importantly, how was I going to lose the eight pounds I gained from eating so much?

However, this experience taught me to be compassionate about women who do get a frightful diagnosis. What if they have children? How will their lives be impacted? No longer am I cavalier about my annual mammogram result. I thank God for a clean report every year.

Since my experience, I've had at least six girlfriends go through the fear of a breast cancer scare. My results were ultimately negative, but some of my friends got positive readings. Knowing what I went through, I give them special care and love because I suspect they, too, are dealing with all the negative thoughts I had about mortality. Most of them run or walk in the Susan G. Komen annual race. I donate and cheer them on. We sisters have to stick together. Negative or positive, the results are never ho hum.

Sharon Hill lives in Chapel Hill, North Carolina with her husband, Elmer Hill. As President of Sharon Hill International, her etiquette training and motivational speaking business, she can be reached at www.sharonhillinternational.com.

A Sprinkle of FUN from Tammy...

Whatever women must do they must do twice as well as men to be thought half as good. Luckily, this is not difficult.

Four Years and Counting: Getting My Life Back
Carol L. Hodes

I can't remember life untouched by cancer. My mother was diagnosed with cancer when I was 12 and, after aggressive treatment, survived for several decades. Not as fortunate, my younger sister was diagnosed with Hodgkin's lymphoma at age 17 and died just before her 22nd birthday. Both of my other siblings have had bouts with various types of cancer. Although I come from a "cancer family", I thought it could not happen to me.

My odyssey began with a routine mammogram in June of 2006, followed by a diagnostic mammogram the next month to examine a suspicious cluster of calcifications. A biopsy was ordered and the radiologist told me that "most of these things are benign—they're nothing." This was followed by a stereotactic biopsy in early September where the radiologist could not penetrate the breast to extract diagnostic samples, so I scheduled an appointment to have a needle-guided surgical biopsy (lumpectomy), a breast conserving technique that uses a barb-ended needle that can only be removed surgically; this procedure removed two large sections of my left breast.

I hoped that the surgical biopsy was the end, not the beginning, but the doctor's call on my cell phone during a 2-hour commute home would prove me wrong. When the doctor said "lobular carcinoma," I pulled over to the side of the road. He continued to say that there was a lot of it, a large amount of abnormal tissue called ductile cancer in situ (DCIS), clear margins had not been achieved, and there was a small area of lobular cancer.

Thoughts of planning the course of treatment seemed frightening and overwhelming. Ten days after the surgical biopsy, my husband and I met my surgical oncologist for about an hour and a half. He was optimistic that my cancer had been detected at a very early stage, but to be safe, he recommended a total mastectomy for at least the left breast. He explained that when my condition was found on one breast, there was a high probability it

161

was on the other side. I was hesitant to accept the most radical approach of a double mastectomy since I had no way to know the extent of the cancer and how much of the breast was involved. Somehow I wanted my diagnosis to be more concrete—something I could see for myself on an x-ray. An option was to do another section of tissue, and if there was not much involvement, have 5-7 weeks of radiation (which has risks of its own).

In early December, my husband, daughter, and I went to Pittsburgh for another opinion. I saw two doctors, an oncologist and a surgical oncologist. They were very pleased that my small local breast center detected an early cancer. The Pittsburgh doctors added to the spectrum of treatment options: one doctor said that I needed five years of an estrogen blocker, such as Evista or Tamoxifen, and the other doctor felt that I needed a round of radiation, but no more surgery. Both doctors impressed upon me that I would always be a breast cancer patient, as if telling me I would undergo a change in identity.

My doctor at home did not agree with the Pittsburgh doctors; he still recommended a total mastectomy based on the large amount of abnormal tissue. I had three different doctors with three opinions! The option with the best long-term prognosis certainly seemed to be the best way to go. I decided I didn't want to take any new drugs and wanted to minimize risk of long-term side effects. Fortunately, as soon as I received my diagnosis, I connected with a support group near my job. Although my own experience has shown that no two cases are identical, I found comfort in sharing the feelings of fear and uncertainty and the group was also an excellent source of information.

The support group also put the positive spin on things to keep the newly diagnosed gals laughing. Benefits of chemo were a free Brazilian wax and not having to shave your legs. I learned where to get the best wigs and even figured out who was wearing one. We had speakers who taught relaxation and ways to pamper ourselves.

My left mastectomy and sentinel node sampling was scheduled for January 2007. The surgery went well and my lymph nodes were negative for cancer. My older daughter, who is a BS, RN and a surgical nurse, was able to stay with me for a few days, which was just wonderful; she took me to the mall for some "retail therapy".

Once the staples and drain were out, arduous physical therapy began; my mobility was only in the 10th percentile by the time I arrived in the physical therapists office! Following with exercises at home, I regained 95% of my range of motion after about 8 weeks. Everyone said that the incision looked good (I think they were just trying to make me feel better), but when you look at yourself in the mirror for the first time, you just cry. It's a big, big adjustment. Being fitted with a prosthesis was a real boost to my emotions; I looked and felt normal again.

On Mother's Day 2007, I braved the crowds and rain to participate in Pittsburgh's "Race For a Cure" with my daughter. I noticed how weak my arms were—I could barely lift anything. When I returned home, I noticed an ad for a cancer wellness program, which I joined. The wellness program was a wonderful opportunity for regaining muscle strength and that last bit of mobility. I worked on weight machines with a trainer to gradually build arm and core strength. I went from lifting 20 to 40 pounds in a few months! I also attended a yoga class with several of the cancer patients and their family members. It's amazing how I always slept better on the nights after yoga. Physical therapy and an ongoing exercise program are a real key to recovery and getting your life back. The good thing about exercise is that it's never too late to start.

I retired in December of 2008 and thought life had returned to normal. However, in January 2011, exactly four years after my mastectomy, I was reminded that I am still and always will be a breast cancer patient, just like the doctors in Pittsburgh said. After a diagnostic mammogram of the right breast, I received news that the changes in calcifications were indicating lobular carcinoma. The doctor said, "Most of these are benign." I am going down that road again.

Carol Hodes lives in State College, PA with her husband, Ron. Dr. Hodes is a retired Sr .Research Associate and maintains an active consulting career through her affiliations with NOCTI and the National Research Center for Career Technical Education. She has two grown daughters and four grandchildren and can be reached at clh4@psualum.com.

A Sprinkle of FUN from Tammy...

"Laughter sometimes out of very private tears."
-- Joan Rivers

My Journey
Patrizia Hoffman

When I was 42 years old, my husband and I left California for Pennsylvania so I could attend grad school at Penn State University. Things were going well until one day, as I was showering, I felt a lump on the side of my left breast. I knew I had never felt it before and wondered how it had developed so quickly. I contacted my OB/GYN to arrange a mammogram. (I had my first one at 40 and it was normal).

The mammogram showed a suspicious lump, so I went for a fine needle aspiration to extract some fluid to be analyzed. The results were inconclusive, and the next step was to have a biopsy done. The surgeon told me that the lump was cancer. After the shock and the numbness had taken hold, I said, "What do we do next?"

Through that hazy time of disbelief and confusion, I had a lumpectomy and waited for the results of my lymph node involvement. Out of a sample of 20 lymph nodes, none were cancerous. I started to feel that I could survive this thing. I had radiation for six weeks and chemotherapy for six months. Throughout this journey, my husband was by my side, coming with me to every treatment and bringing me back and forth to my classes and teaching responsibilities at Penn State.

During my treatment I found out about Reach to Recovery (RTR) from a friend who had been diagnosed six months before me and had been visited by an RTR volunteer. As soon as I heard about what the RTR volunteers did, I knew that I wanted to do the same for other women. I trained with Betty Blackadar who was a 20-year survivor when I met her in State College.

I loved having the opportunity to visit with newly diagnosed women to let them know I had been through breast cancer and survived. I felt that every year I lived I was an inspiration and role model for others to believe that they too can survive.

When I moved to Clinton County eight years ago, I signed up to be a local RTR volunteer. Today, I am blessed to say that I am an 18 year and 9 month survivor of breast cancer.

Patrizia Hoffman is a Professor of Communication at Lock Haven University of PA and lives in a Victorian era home with her husband of 45 years, Fredrick, and their three Westies - Tricky Woo, Benny Woo and Bonnie.

A Sprinkle of FUN from Tammy…

"Life is uncertain, eat your dessert first!"
Credited to a lot of people, but I think my mother, Ruth Miller, is the original author!

More Open to Love
Susan R. Holderman

I was diagnosed with breast cancer on February 23rd, 2011. My doctor called at 4:51 PM, just as I was arriving home from work. I remember it vividly as I had a daily date at 5:00 to run with a friend. Funny, but I was more concerned about holding up my run than what was actually being told to me. "Blah blah, cancer, blah blah, refer you to Dr. blah, blah..." I thanked him for calling, but deep down I knew what was happening long before the call. I knew my body and I knew that this lump felt differently than the two I had found 4 years earlier. I already had a lumpectomy and 3 benign tumors removed from both breasts. I allowed myself to cry a few tears at the thought of telling my 17-year-old daughter who had lost her great grandmother a month earlier to cancer. I did not want to have to say the 'c' word to her again. Quickly I called her father; we have been divorced for 10 years. I asked that he be on the same page and to put on a brave front should she come to him. I made another quick call to a friend who had anxiously awaited the results of the most recent biopsy and then it was off for my run.

Until this point I was a single mom, raising my daughter and niece while working two jobs to make ends meet. When I heard the cancer diagnosis, my first thought was "what a relief." Odd feeling, breathing a sigh of relief after being told you have breast cancer, but for the first time in years I allowed myself to slow down and not feel so pressured. I had a good excuse to take time to take care of myself. Not once do I remember feeling fear. I was confident that the cancer was detected early, and as I would find out many mammograms, MRI's and biopsies later, it had not spread. Yet another blessing, the cancer was ER (estrogen receptor) positive and would respond well to adjuvant therapy with Tamoxifen as opposed to chemo or radiation after my surgery.

Due to the size of the tumor and previous lumpectomies, I knew that my best course of action would be to have a prophylactic bilateral mastectomy. This may seem radical to some when

167

genetic testing for the BRCA 1 & 2 genes came back negative. However, I only needed to hear "you have cancer" once in my life. The thought of even one more lumpectomy for a benign mass was more than I wanted to endure. I was relieved that my surgeon was on board and supported my decision. She arranged for her group's plastic surgeon to perform the reconstruction at the same time.

The surgery to remove all subcutaneous breast tissue but preserve skin and the nipple, although painful, went smoothly. Expanders, temporary implants inserted under remaining tissue, were put in and filled at regular intervals over the next month and a half until the desired volume was obtained; I currently have them in. They are hard, uncomfortable, and hurt a little after each filling, but they will be removed in two to three months and replaced with silicone implants with a more natural look and feel.

I was referred to a local oncologist for aftercare and prescribed Tamoxifen daily for the next five years to prevent new breast cancers from developing. Oncotype testing estimated my risk of reoccurrence at only 9% but I like the added 'insurance policy' it provided. I was very lucky compared to what some other women go through during treatment; I felt embarrassed to even say I was a survivor because my treatment was fast and relatively easy. So much so, that just two weeks after surgery I was schlepping it up the side of Hyner Mountain at their annual 20K Trail run that I had signed up for back in January. My boyfriend encouraged me to hike as much as I could, and his sister in law, my dear friend, questioned my decision as she helped me pin on my racing number. I made it 3.5 miles that day - not the full 14.6 miles I had been training for but quite a victory for me! Please, do not tell my doctor! He did not recommend this although part of me thinks he would be pleased too!

I look back now, almost 3 months from diagnosis, and am impressed at how well I handled the situation. Not that I didn't get frustrated or down; I remember one time that I was feeling a bit overwhelmed. My dad was my rock in life and I visit his gravesite when I need him. I remember sitting there, crying about what I was going through and the challenges I faced when I heard his voice in my head saying, "Suz, look around you." I was sitting in a field of stone, people who would never have a chance at another tomorrow. Ever try to host a pity party in a cemetery? It's a very humbling experience!

I also credit my faith in God for giving me the strength that I needed the moment the doctor called. If it weren't for Him and the peace He provided to me, I would have lost it from the strain of an already stressful life. He blessed me with loving friends and family who assisted and cared for me during my recovery. I was overwhelmed with the love I felt and eternally grateful for the phone calls, outings, prepared meals and other blessings that found their way to me.

A very dear friend was there for me and my girls during the surgery and I was so glad to have them by my side that day! I'm dating a loving, nurturing guy who made me dinner, helped me shower, and provided me with that little kick in the butt I needed from time to time. He made me feel beautiful although I wasn't always feeling it myself. For most women, their breasts are a very large part of their sexuality. This was very true for me but my boyfriend would remind me how superficial that was with "baby we are talking about your health." He was right, and now we laugh at the 80's bad porn boob job looking appearance of the expanders and him drumming on a very rigid saline expander filled breast.

I've laughed more than I've cried, and those tears were often happy tears. Instead of waiting for friends to come to me, I became the friend I wanted to have. I found myself reaching out more to the people in my life. Shouldn't I have been more upset? Often times I thought maybe I was in denial over the whole process but all I can see when I look back over my journey are the blessings that I have received. I am closer to God, I am more open to love, I have learned to appreciate the people in my life a little more, and I just do not have tears for the cancer, the pain, or the scars I will carry for life.

Susan lives in Bellefonte, PA with her daughter, Sarah and niece, Lena. She maintains a healthy and active lifestyle which she attributes much of her healing success to and has competed in 4 trail run races ranging from a 4.3 mile, clothing optional race (which she was proud to bear her scars for and benefiting the cancer society of course) to an 18.9 mile race in the 10 weeks since her surgery. She challenges women living with cancer to see the hope and find the strength within themselves as well.

A Sprinkle of FUN from Tammy...

"Whoever thought up the word "Mammogram"? Every time I hear it, I think I'm supposed to put my breast in an envelope and send it to someone."   -- Jan King

Self-Exam, My Life Saver
Cindy Holobusky

Five years ago I discovered a lump on my breast. I had just taken a shower when I did my self-exam. My husband felt it wasn't anything to worry about. I felt a need to call my doctor right away. He told me to come right in, then he checked me; that's when he also felt the lump. Afterwards, he sent me to get some tests done.

A week later, I got a phone call from the doctor's office to come in because he wanted to talk to me. I took my best friend Dorothy with me, thinking maybe it wasn't anything. Well I was wrong; the news was that I had breast cancer. When I was given the news, all I could think of was that I was going to die. Why? Because I had lost my mother at the age of forty-eight (I was only in my twenty's) on Christmas day to cancer. Her death was due to another type of cancer. So to me, the word cancer meant death.

I was only forty-six and had my life ahead of me. I had just gotten remarried and we were planning on buying a home. My oncologist told me to go ahead and buy that home. He did promise to take very good care of me, because I had some other health conditions. He was very nervous because he had to talk with some of my doctors. I have had three major heart operations. The first one was at the age of eight, then the second one at the age of forty, and the third one at the age of forty-three. At the age of forty-six, I was told that I had breast cancer. My oncologist had to work very close with my cardiologist, knowing that I had two artificial heart valves, and that I needed to stay out of any danger because I was taking a blood thinner. I was very terrified that I had to have another operation.

My doctors all did a wonderful job. I appreciate them so much for all their care, patience, kindness, and understanding. I'll never forget saying to my oncologist, "Thank-you for taking such good care of me."

His answer back was, "No Cindy, let me say thank-you for allowing me to take care of you; it was an honor." Today, I'm a five-year survivor of breast cancer. I truly believe I saved my own

171

life, by doing the self-exam and making that phone call to my doctor. I'm a firm believer in making sure all women do the self-exams. The mammogram never discovered my lump; I did.

Cindy lives in Walnutport, PA with her wonderful husband of eight years, Brian. She has a wonderful daughter, Megan, who is 23, and a wonderful son, Will who is 15. They both mean the world to her. She works at a daycare, which she loves very much because the children are so special. She enjoys reading, going for walks, playing cards and doing puzzles. She also loves to give back to others in any way that she can and she appreciates working with the American Heart Association, and the PA Breast Cancer Coalition, who allow her to do this.

Sisters
Teresa Homan

Cindy and I were sisters. We were born two years apart. We had the same parents. We lived under the same roof. Cindy and I were sisters, but you would never know it. Aside from the fact that we shared the same parents and the same household during our childhood, Cindy and I were not close. We were not the sisters that stayed up all night talking after our mother told us to turn out the lights. We were not the sisters who chose to attend nearby colleges. We were not the sisters who started our own families and made sure to move into the same neighborhood. We were sisters, but we were not close. That is, until I was diagnosed with breast cancer.

My battle with breast cancer began in September of 2001. Over the next few months, I kept returning to the doctor, needing to have a lump in my breast removed. Although I never needed to undergo any chemotherapy or radiation treatment, I ultimately had a mastectomy in February of 2002. From my first operation in September until my full recovery and start of survivorship in 2004, Cindy was by my side.

Throughout my battle, I always kept a positive attitude. I knew that this was something that just had to be taken care. I would deal with it now and be done with it. I also kept telling myself: if I can get through this, I can get through anything. But the most important part of maintaining this positive attitude was to surround myself with positive people. My husband, Mick, was right by my side starting with that first lumpectomy. But, I had expected that from him. Mick had always been my rock and I knew that he would stay positive with me through this next challenge in my life. In my sister Cindy though, I found an unexpected companion. Cindy was there to cheer me up on days I was feeling down. She brought a womanly understanding to the whole experience. And Cindy was not only there for me, she was there for Mick as well.

Around the time of my surgery in February, I heard that an old classmate of mine from high school had been diagnosed with breast cancer as well. Unlike my cancer though, which was stage zero, her cancer was caught at a rather advanced stage. She fought a long, courageous battle, but ultimately, the cancer took her life. Throughout the rest of my own treatment, I used faith and prayer to keep me going. But suddenly, I questioned, why had God spared me?

I firmly believe that everything happens for a reason. Although we don't always understand why things happen the way they do, God has a reason. After surviving my battle, I chose to change career paths. I was so grateful to the many nurses and doctors who had been there for me that I wanted to give back to the medical community. I went back to school and today, I work in an oncology office. It offers me a one on one opportunity with cancer patients that are going through what I have gone through. I can share with them my stories and also my positive attitude. I am there to tell them- "Hey, I've been here. I've done that. And I am standing here in front of you today. You can get through this."

I feel very blessed that God spared my life and for the reasons he did it. Every day I feel blessed for the new career I have and for the many connections I make with patients. I feel blessed that God brought me closer to the sister I always should have had. Breast cancer totally changed my life, but I know that God had my life change for a reason.

Throughout the reconstructive stages of my treatment, I found it most important to find the humor in everything. During the summer of 2003, my husband and I made a trip to the beach. I had begun my reconstructive surgery and had little feeling around my breast. Besides the numbness around my breast, I remember the water was so cold that the rest of my body was numb as well. Mick and I were having a blast in the water, when a few waves headed our way. I managed to remain standing as they passed, thinking I made out pretty well by not falling. "Uh, hunny.." Mick said, trying to get my attention. It was at that moment that I realized I was facing my fellow beach goers, completely topless.

The water had not only made me lose feeling in my body, it had made me lose my bathing suit top as well! "Well," I said, "at least no one can tell that they aren't real- I just had my nipple tattoos done!" Mick and I both started laughing. At my next doctor's appointment, I told my plastic surgeon he should thank me. "For what?" he asked. I told him that I had given him free advertising at the beach! Everyone got an eyeful of his fabulous work!

Today, as I reach 7 years of survivorship, Cindy and I remain close. Although we do not live close enough to see each other often, we talk on the phone once a week. We think about each other all the time. Whenever I am shopping and see something with that signature pink breast cancer ribbon, I make sure to buy two- one for myself and one for Cindy. Cindy does the same for me. T-shirts, plates, ornaments, you name it. It is our little way to let each other know that we are thinking of each other. It is our way to let each other know we are thankful for the other's friendship.

Cindy and I are sisters, and now, I really truly believe you would know it.

Teresa Homan
As written by Taryn Noll

Teresa lives in Shippensurg, PA with her husband Mick and their 5 dogs. She works for a Urology office in Camp Hill, PA. You can reach her at teresahoman6@centurylink.net

I Believe
Terry Hood

I was diagnosed with breast cancer in 1991, at the age of 33, while nursing my youngest daughter. I felt a lump under my arm, which was thought to be from mastitis. After a round of antibiotics, and then weaning her, the lump persisted. I had the lymph node removed and was floored to hear "metastatic lymph node, most likely primary, breast." My daughters at the time were young, Elyse was almost 4, Lindsey was 2 1/2, and Ashley was 8 months old. My diagnosis was Stage 3 breast cancer, 7 of 8 lymph nodes were positive, dermal and lymphatic involvement with negative receptors. I underwent a mastectomy, bone marrow harvesting, high dose chemotherapy and radiation.

Everyone who has walked this path has a story. I like to look back now and think of how cancer has changed my life.

I Believe - Cancer is not all bad. Cancer allows you to prioritize differently. Little things that might have bothered you before... don't anymore. You know who and what is important in your life and you may not have time for some of the "small stuff."

I Believe - You meet wonderful people while walking this walk. From the family and friends that you already count on, you then meet doctors, nurses, support people and a huge new family of women who know exactly how you feel and can relate to you. They become sisters to you, and you to them.

I Believe - Your attitude plays a huge part in your treatment. As hard as it sometimes may be, keeping a positive attitude and trying to see things in that light, helps.

I Believe - I believe that there is definitely a place for support groups. Whether a person feels like participating in an actual group, or just mentors to someone who is going through the same thing, is huge. All of us have so much to share, and every one of the women diagnosed need to know they have someone to talk to.

I am a twenty year survivor now! When I was diagnosed I wasn't sure I would see my girls start kindergarten, and I am proud to say two have graduated from college and my youngest is finishing her nursing degree now. In twenty years I have seen huge progress made in this field. We need to keep supporting the cause, as much and as often as we can.

Thank you and God Bless,
Terry Hood

Terry is from Conneaut Lake, PA and works at her community hospital as an ultrasound technologist and has worked there for over 25 years. She and her husband are the parents to three beautiful daughters.

Don't Tilt the Canoe
Donna Lee Irwin

When I was first diagnosed, I just sat there and said "Okay, what now?" This shocked my doctor, since this is not the typical reaction women have when they hear they have breast cancer. I was just very calm about the whole situation, the calmest out of everyone around me.

At the time, I lived with my daughter Lisa and also my parents. My parents were living with me temporarily. They had just finished up their traveling and we were looking into getting them out on their own again. Then, I was diagnosed, and they knew they needed to stick around to help. My mom was wonderful, being the mom that she is. And my dad, who lost his hair at age 19, helped me through the trauma of losing my long hair, with much humor and camaraderie.

My daughter Lisa burst into tears at the news of my diagnosis. She was twenty years old, always dressed in black and had hair that flowed down her back. After the news, Lisa shocked the world and me. She started wearing pink. She donated her long, flowing hair. She turned into a great cheerleader for me. It was Lisa's great sense of humor that helped me get through it all. I will never forget the time we were in the mastectomy boutique. Lisa started throwing the prosthetics around and was trying on all the wigs. I was laughing so hard. I can only imagine what the owners of the store thought, but I knew Lisa didn't care. She was just acting goofy and making me laugh, and that was all that mattered to her.

As I made the decision about my mastectomy, my daughter and my best friend Kevin used their humor to weigh in on this situation as well. I could not decide whether I should have both breasts removed or not. Lisa simply said, "Mom, you are going to be 45 years old. Why have one perky 25 year old boob? Just get both done." Kevin simply said, I had better even them out soon so we don't keep tilting to one side while canoeing. Lisa and I were always very close, but her humor and support throughout my treatment brought us even closer together as mother and daughter.

During my treatment, I didn't take any time off of work. I work at a family chiropractic office in Latrobe, Pennsylvania. At home, my parents, my daughter and my boyfriend Jesse were all doing an amazing job of supporting me, and at work, this was no different. My boss, the receptionist Ellen, and Vicki, the other massage therapist were truly amazing. Vicki organized an entire benefit for me. She knew that I was supporting myself and my daughter, all while battling breast cancer. The benefit had hundreds of people attend; even some of the patients from our office came. My boss, Dr. Dave, was especially supportive. On the night of my mastectomy, he spent the night with me in the hospital. Slept on a chair in my room all night, just to be there for me.

The most supportive of all was my best friend Luanne. She was with me from the very beginning, attending each and every Dr.'s appointment, and sitting through every single chemo treatment that lasted 6 hours, never once leaving my side. She has been my rock and continues to be there for me 24/7.

I did not miss much work. I felt that if I let myself sit at home, it would all hit me. I did not need to be sitting around thinking about it. I needed to stay positive and move on. On days when I was off from work though, my co-workers kept a journal in the office. It was here that they wrote their thoughts and prayers to me. Anytime in my life when I think I am not loved, I pull that book out and read what people wrote. These people were truly unbelievable to me.

The patients think I am so chipper and happy nowadays, even during my treatment. To be honest though, I feel the cancer has been a gift, as odd as it sounds. Because of breast cancer I am doing many of things I've always wanted to do, but never took the time to. I am reading everything and have had a major lifestyle change. When I was diagnosed, I found the urge to dive into holistic health. I focused on different ways to make the body resistant to cancers. I'm sure my daughter got a little sick of me telling what she could and could not eat. I did get a little crazy with it, analyzing every single food and substance that could cause cancer. But now, I get to teach classes on using nutrition, exercise and natural therapies as cancer prevention. I can listen to these patients and I can sympathize with them. Hopefully, I can help them, because I've been there. In fact, I am still there. Right now, I am in the very last stages of radiation. I was so burnt that I had to stop for two weeks. Of course, I continued working.

Everyone calls me an inspiration. Really though, I am not. Before my diagnosis, I wasn't appreciating life for what it is. Now, I love each day, because each day is a gift. Breast cancer motivated me to do what I have talked about doing for years. Everything happens for a reason and I truly believe this in my heart. Breast cancer has been an incredible journey and I wouldn't change a thing about it. I have learned about the generosity of people. I look back now and see all that I have learned, and continue to learn, and I feel more blessed now than ever.

Donna Lee Irwin
As written by Taryn Noll

Donna Lee Irwin is a Certified Massage Therapist who works at Deglau Family Chiropractic in Latrobe, PA. She currently is living in Derry, PA with her family, and is training with the American Cancer Society as a counselor, while doing massage and teaching health and wellness classes at the chiropractic clinic. Donna Lee can be reached at silvermusicwoman@yahoo.com.

My Pink Ribbon Story
Jeanne Itak

I was "officially" diagnosed with stage II breast cancer on Dec. 21, 2009. I held off telling my children and family until after Christmas Day and spent my "vacation" between Christmas and New Years at the hospital and radiology center fully staging the disease with CT Scans, MRIs, PET Scan and bones scans. I kicked off 2010 by getting my infusion port inserted into my arm and a few days later started what would become a 6 month chemotherapy regimen. Once I had embarked on my treatment plan, my thoughts turned more to worrying about the impact of my disease on my 2 teenage daughters. My younger daughter, Sara, was home and I could keep an eye on her. My other daughter, Kelsey, had just finished her first semester as a freshman at Penn State University (PSU) and was headed back to school by mid-January. I was concerned how she would cope.

Shortly after returning for her spring semester, Kelsey told us she had joined a new club that was forming at PSU focused on breast cancer awareness called The Power of Pink. At first I thought how great it was that she had found a support group who could help her, but she has shown her intentions to be more unselfish and philanthropic. Initially, she had planned to organize a team of family members to participate in the Philadelphia Race for the Cure in the spring. Unfortunately, this occurred during Mother's Day weekend, right around the time I was finishing up my chemotherapy and I did not have the energy to participate. Undeterred, she volunteered to co-chair the club's inaugural fundraising race scheduled for October, 2010.

Preliminary race planning began that semester but really kicked into high gear when Kelsey returned to school in August. In addition to her sizable class workload, a board position on her business club and busy social life, she worked tirelessly to make the race a success. She solicited numerous local businesses to be sponsors to donate food and water, she designed the race trophies, collaborated on advertising and recruitment at the college and surrounding communities to attract participants and coordinated with other club members to bring the event details together.

The Sunday morning of the race was a beautiful fall day. Stephen, my husband, Sara and I traveled to PSU with my mother, Cynthia, a 14 year survivor and the oldest participant. We arrived to find Kelsey and her friends hard at work setting up the race area. It was amazing! They had tents for registration, food and water. They provided information and cross-promoted other breast cancer events with other PSU groups like the women's basketball Pink Zone game. Deejays from a local radio station were on hand playing music and getting the crowd excited. A giant finish line had been erected and everywhere there were pink balloons. The club had hoped to attract 100 participants to their first annual event but everyone was overwhelmed to have over 200 registrants by race time.

Looking back, I'm not sure what I liked best about the day: the pride in seeing what my daughter made happen, crossing the finish line with my 78 year old mother or the joy I felt in knowing that what had happened to me had not weakened Kelsey but had empowered her and made her stronger. She has chosen to make a difference and be part of the solution to finding a cure. She continues this work. She is a truly remarkable young woman.

Jeanne lives with her husband, two daughters and 3 pugs in NJ. She works for Johnson & Johnson and in her free time enjoys the beach, photography and puzzles. Her daughter is also one of the "Pink Ribbon Writers" for this book.

My Inspiration
Kelsey Itak

I was home for Christmas break during my freshman year of college. One night my dad, almost sounding angry, called my younger sister and me downstairs. I walked into the living room to see my mom on the couch, eyes red and puffy, and my dad looking solemn as ever. "We have something to tell you," he said. The next 10 seconds seemed like an eternity, as I had a million thoughts run through my mind. Did someone die? Did one of my parents lose their job? My mom then burst into tears whispering, "I can't. I can't do it." Becoming extremely concerned, I looked at my dad for something; anything to end this suspense. "Mom has cancer," he said bluntly. I remember the silence that engulfed the room; I stared at him, then looked at my mom, speechless for a minute. She regained her composure and stated, "I'm fine. Women are diagnosed with breast cancer all the time. Really, everything is going to work out." Incredibly, that was the attitude she kept throughout the following months.

When I returned to Penn State, I had a hard time dealing with the fact that my mom would be starting treatment and I was 200 miles away with no idea what was happening. At first, I didn't talk to anyone about it, and tried to continue with school as though everything was normal. I figured if people knew, they would ask me how I was doing all the time and that would make the whole situation more difficult for me. After a while, though, I needed some sort of outlet and decided to confide in my closest friend, Sean. Talking to her helped me more than I ever could have imagined. Much of the time, she would just listen and assure me that if anyone could beat this cancer, it was my mom. She seemed so certain that everything would work out, and that certainty is what ultimately structured my optimistic perspective throughout the rest of my mom's battle.

I began getting frustrated with my mother, though, because every time I would call to see how she was doing, she would reply with, "Good. How's school going? How are classes?" I assumed that she wanted to seem upbeat so that I wouldn't be worrying about her all the time, but it almost made me more concerned because I never knew what was going on. Luckily, Sean told me about someone she knew who was trying to start a breast cancer club at school. Taryn, another freshman, was working with Susan G. Komen to form an on-campus organization to help raise money and awareness for breast cancer research. Her mom was diagnosed about a month before mine, so I felt that this was the perfect opportunity for me to make a friend who was dealing with the same things, as well as help the cause. Taryn was truly an inspiration. Her positive attitude and determination for the success of the club was incredible. After talking to her about my own situation, she asked me to take the position as Race Chair for the club, The Power of Pink. Of course, I gladly accepted! My responsibilities included organizing our inaugural 5K on campus, seeking sponsorship, and creating strategies to involve, not only Penn State students, but also the local community.

Meanwhile, back at home, my mom was struggling with one obstacle after another to beat her cancer; for a while it seemed as though there was no end in sight. She went through 5 months of chemotherapy, a double-mastectomy, and then was told that she would need 28 rounds of radiation. It was a grueling year, but all of her strength and determination helped her overcome it.

On the day of the race for The Power of Pink, everything went perfectly. After months of treatment, my mom was able to run as a survivor! My whole family came, including my grandmother who is a 14-year survivor herself. The weather was beautiful and every aspect of the event seemed to fall right into place. We ended up with over 200 race participants, far surpassing our initial goal of 100. All of the club members were there to assist with set-up, food and water donations, and distributing numbers and timers for the runners. It was amazing to see so many people working together for this cause. At the end of the day, we found out that the event raised nearly $4,000, an unbelievable feat.

Not long after the race, I was presented with the opportunity to work with Taryn on this book, Pink Ribbon Stories.

Tammy Miller, the author, is another inspiration who displays an eternally optimistic outlook on life. I was eager to join the book team, especially because the purpose was to collect stories "to encourage, inspire, and make you smile." While working on this book, I have met all kinds of incredible women. From the other people I'm working with, to the ones that I interviewed, I have constantly been amazed by the sincerity and positive attitudes expressed by each and every woman I spoke with.

Now, more than a year after my mom's diagnosis, it is evident that my friends, the Power of Pink members, and this book team have helped me with much more than just dealing with my mom's disease. After realizing how many people are coping with the same situation, (and there are a lot,) I am not so quick to make judgments when someone is displaying a bitter attitude. I understand that you should offer support rather than annoyance because you have no idea what emotional or physical difficulties they could be facing.

My mom battled her cancer with strength, determination, and poise. The obstacles she was forced to overcome were unimaginable, and she conquered them without ever stopping to take a breath. She was incredible throughout everything, and I am so unbelievably proud of her. I believe that everything I've been involved with over the past year has shaped me in several profound and important ways. I feel that it has made me a stronger, more compassionate person, and I hope that makes me mom just as proud of me.

Kelsey is currently a junior at Penn State. She is from West Windsor, NJ, where her parents, sister, and 3 pugs all live. Kelsey is one of the Pink Ribbon Writers for this book.

Why Wait?
Donna James

Pink was never a favourite colour of mine – it still isn't. But for me, and the rest of the world -- pink is now more than just a colour …it's a powerful brand that implies much more than soft and pretty "girly" stuff. PINK is now universally-recognized, not as a representation of passive feminine influence, but as a symbol of the extraordinary strength that can be gained from dealing with a life-threatening diagnosis.

Significant change is always born of strong emotion. Even if you haven't been faced with breast cancer, there is probably some sort of event that changed your life in a similar way… something that took your breath away when it happened,… something that reduced the universe to a space that was, for a while, only large enough for you and your fear.

In October of 1993, my life was finally feeling like it was back within my control. For the past 18 months I had juggled the care of my dying mother, the needs of my family, and my full time job – a lot of you know exactly what that's like – you never feel that you are doing a great job of any of them --- someone or something always seems to be needing more than you have to give – the guilt is unrelenting.

It had been 5 months since my mother had lost her battle with breast cancer, and I was beginning to get my old life back – back on automatic pilot, filling up my days and nights with the old "busy-ness", filling up my body with the old diet -- coffee, cigarettes and junk food ---, and unconsciously going through all those day-to-day activities with no time for self-examination, or any true appreciation of my blessings. Looking back on it today, it's easy to see how circumstances conspired to bring me to my senses.

It was a normal yearly mammogram – and although it came on the heels of my mother's death, it didn't really scare me.

It was the last time I was ever going to feel that way.

Even when the doctor at the radiology lab told me that a "suspicious calcification" had appeared on my film, by that time I'd had so many unusual images on my mammograms, so many aspirated lumps and indeterminate "thickenings", that it had no special significance for me. Besides, I was on the tamoxifen drug trial, and every small change was very significant, so even when a biopsy was scheduled, I viewed it in the context of overly-cautious research.

I remember saying to my niece just before my biopsy ..." If this turns out badly, I think I'll probably become very involved in this cause."

I realize now that I was pretty cavalier at that point; it was easy, then, to be noble. I had done door-to-door canvassing every year after my mother was diagnosed, never seriously considering the implications for my own health. My approach to the threat had always been pretty unemotional... I had even decided that when my cancer was discovered, I would opt for a lumpectomy, and maybe a little chemo "chaser".... like a buffet I'd just breeze through and be done with. At that point having cancer in my own body never felt like a real possibility...

From time to time I pull out the Daytimer page from October 21, 1993, just to remind myself of how quickly a life can change. On that page is written... "1PM – Surgeon/results ... 2PM - Back to office". I didn't get back to the office for over a week – and in that week I was transported to an alternate reality, as I made plans for a mastectomy and talked to my family in terms of how they would have to function after I was gone.

Alone with the enormous grief, anger, and disbelief that comes with a diagnosis, your first thoughts are normally far from constructive. Getting out of the "ground zero tape loop" is one of the toughest parts. You know the "ground zero" tape --- the one where all of your senses combine to create a moment so surreal that you have to play and replay it, because there must be a glitch in there somewhere that will reveal it as simply a huge misunderstanding. --

After the mastectomy, the pathology was encouraging –
clear margins, no nodes affected – Stage Zero …thanks to the
tamoxifen trial I was part of, they had caught it exceptionally early.
(Note: If you ever get the chance to take part in a drug trial, do it.
Even if it turns out that you are on the control group taking a
placebo, as I was, you'll never have better care, or a better chance
of early intervention.)

During the first months after my surgery, I was simply
driven. Using reserves of energy I had never tapped before --
although I didn't understand that at the time – I plowed ahead.
Creating a positive change for those touched by breast cancer, once
an idle promise… was now a real passion. I often refer to my
whole cancer experience as part of God's "Catch and Release"
Program. You re-prioritize very quickly.

My husband and I sold our business, we both found ways to
make a living doing things we really enjoyed, and started devoting
lots of time to the leisure activities we loved as well.

I had always enjoyed volunteering, so I began to devote a
much larger part of my life to breast cancer charities.

Don't delude yourself. Volunteerism is a purely selfish
pursuit. There is nothing more enjoyable than giving yourself to
something that makes life better for a whole lot of people. The
bigger the community return the better. And it's good for you.
Anecdotal evidence suggests that volunteers live longer lives …
something to do with the connection between happiness and the
immune system….

My need for emotional support was first met by the
survivors within the group therapy program at our local cancer care
facility, but having given up my 35-year smoking habit, I was 30
pounds heavier and in need of some help.

One day in 1997, I heard about an exciting sport that had
been "making waves" off the west coast for a couple of years –
survivor dragon boat racing. I helped to establish a team in my
own city – and it got me hooked for life on the benefits of regular
physical activity.

I have a full and wonderful life, and I try not to take any of it for granted – things can change in a heartbeat. Then it's important to remember that your misfortunes can provide some of the greatest gifts in your life – calm seas don't produce great sailors. Just so you don't forget, surround yourself with great people who will remind you.

I want to finish off by giving you a little exercise you can perform to keep yourself focused. This comes courtesy of Aniko Galambos, a former hard-driving corporate executive, who completely "re-designed" her life after a diagnosis of breast cancer...

"If you found out tomorrow that you had cancer... you would probably make a lot of changes in your life. You would probably start by eliminating all of the toxic elements you've been living with every day-- be they foods, or people, or unhealthy behaviours. You would also begin to embrace more of the things that bring you joy and strength.

My question to you is this: ... "Why wait?"

Donna James lives happily in Edmonton, Alberta with her husband, Keith. She is helping to build a cancer support and wellness centre called, Wellspring, and has a thriving business called Wooly Boulevard, making felted jewelry both online and at local artisan fairs.

Hold My Calls, Please
Kathy Julian

God has a funny way of answering prayers.

When my Mom got sick, she prayed, fervently, that my family (my husband, myself and my recently married daughter, Erika) would move home. Amazingly, God provided an awesome job opportunity for my husband and my daughter's recent "marriage" was a reality check and eye opener. She followed us 6 months later.

On a hospital "visit," the emergency doctor that examined Mom asked my sister and me how long she'd had breast cancer…? Our mouths dropped open… We never knew. She said she had felt a lump 15 years ago and just hoped it would go away. That's my Mom. But now it was the size of a golf ball. With her health issues, age and weight (she weighed less than 100 pounds), she refused all treatments, surgery, chemotherapy, etc… We went to the Breast Cancer doctor for a biopsy and were referred to a great specialist, Dr. Raymond, and her assistant, JoAnne.

They had a blood treatment (Herceptin) that sounded like an answer to our prayers. After only the first treatment, however, she went into anaphylactic shock and was hospitalized. She was then put on cancer pills (Tykerb) which, when I went to purchase found out they were $3000! I could have paid it if it was they whole year's supply, but this was just for one month. Dr. Raymond called the drug company and they graciously sent her the prescription for $35 per month. Big difference! The pills were large and she had to take 4 every day, but she took them. She'd say she had "a meal" of pills. There were quite a few, and with her other ailments, it did make a meal! She wasn't a big eater anyway. I complained to her all the time. She watched a lot of television and would forget to eat.

She would get up early, watch church on television, then have breakfast, and then accept phone calls (you couldn't call during church!). Then there were the game shows (35 year-old reruns!), Judge Judy, Law & Order, Jeopardy! (no phone calls then, either), Wheel of Fortune, etc… Her fingers were so crooked from arthritis that she couldn't do much. She managed to write her checks though. I could have done it for her but she needed to do it. It was good exercise for her hands.

She drove me crazy with her pills though. I would come in one day and ask if there was anything she needed from the store; food, medicine, supplies, etc. No, nothing – or she'd give me a list of things – no problem. I'd say that I had things to do the next day and wouldn't be in, so I wanted to accomplish as much as possible. Then, the very next day, I would call her and she would tell me that she needed her prescription! I would get a little angry because I had just asked her the day before… Then I would tell her, "That pill fairy had better stop stealing your pills!" Sometimes I would go to get her a prescription every other day. I had her birth date and year memorized better than my own!

There were so many plans for the future. I know she met Christopher (her future great-grandson) up in Heaven, but I would have liked to have a photograph of her and the memories of us all together. It wasn't right though, to make her suffer. She wanted to go so much and she begged me every day and every time I was there to let her go. I worry that I will be judged for her death. It's really hard to know that I am to blame; even though we all had to agree, it was me that had to talk with her doctors and start the process. She was happy though, there would be no more pain. I wish we could have seen her with Christopher. She would love him so much. He would be the light of her life, just like Erika was.

It's funny, I would tell her of how she prayed to get us to live closer and how God answered her prayers. Then I would say maybe pray that we hit the lottery or something big like that! I guess really, when you think about it, we did hit the best lottery of all – we had more time and memories to have with my Mom.

Kathy lives in Robinson Township, PA with her husband, Rick, and their 4 rescued cats. She is a stay-at-home grandma who adores spending time with her grandson. She loves sewing and doing crafts of all kinds.

A Journal of Breast Cancer
Betty Kauffman

In April of 1977 I was diagnosed with breast cancer. These are my initial feelings, as written in my journal, as I faced the journey for treatment.

I had heard of many cases of breast cancer in women. I had never, physically, seen the aftermath of a woman who had a mastectomy, but I could imagine the trauma one must go through. You see others, but never believe you may one day be stricken.

I lived in a small town in PA, a young woman in my thirties, healthy, bursting with energy, but one day I was faced with the realization of a sizeable lump in my right breast. After two years of check ups and mammographies, the doctor decided the lump may be malignant.

I was devastated of course and began to search my soul for an answer. I would never have a mastectomy! I would die first! Only a few weeks before this despairing news, my husband had brought to my attention a one page article in Time magazine titled "The Alternative to Mastectomy". The treatment mentioned in the article entailed 30 radiation treatments followed by interstitial implants using isotope iridium 192, threaded through the breast. I clipped it out and put it in my file, never dreaming it might be my only hope.

The doctor recommended the removal of the tumor at once, and of course, a mastectomy. With article in hand, I met with my surgeon and explained my strong feelings and asked for his help. Yes, he had heard of this procedure; however it was not in the medical journal and they did it only in California. Well, California, here I come! Would he please make the arrangements, at my expense, no less? His refusal and his associates' rude remarks pushed me into total depression. Dead end!

I finally approved the removal of the tumor, still hoping, somehow, somewhere I would find hope. The surgery went well. Yes, the tumor was malignant as suspected. Two days later I was home and back to work, stronger now - determined to find a way.

My husband and I scheduled a consultation with another doctor who said, "Well, it might be okay, but I am not interested in helping." Another dead end. Constant phone calls that included: "You can't wait, you must have your breast removed - it's the only way; no one cares if you have only one breast - you can have reconstruction surgery."

I care, it's my body and I CARE! I know me and I cannot accept the fact. I'd rather die.

My husband was very understanding. No, it would not bother him but he knew me and knew that radical surgery would wreck me mentally. I became despondent, screaming at him to do something. He could alleviate most any situation, why not this? Finally, he cut off all the phone calls. Oh, everyone thought they were being helpful, but the mention of mastectomy threw me into nausea and hysteria. It was out of the question. Final as death! I never wanted to hear the word again.

I met with the surgeon again and inquired about going to Bethesda, Md. And still the answer was "No - there was no protocol for people like me!" COULDN'T ANYONE UNDERSTAND?

Finally after two months of total trauma I met with a wonderful and understanding oncologist. He read my now "worn" article and reached for the phone. He got nowhere that day, but promised he would have answers for me within two days. The next afternoon I received his call. It was all there: No it would not be as easy as the article made it sound, but the statistics for radiation implants were every bit as good as radical mastectomies. He was very impressed with the findings and yes, he would recommend it. They were able to do the procedure in Boston!

Before I knew it I was off to Boston to start treatments. My husband and I drove to Boston and met with the head of the radiology department. He explained the procedure. In nine years with this method, he had experienced only one complete failure. They set me up for treatments, putting me through a simulation first.

We drove home and the following Monday I was on a plane to Boston - alone. I had reserved a room in a nearby motel and was all set. I had to stay Monday thru Friday getting treatment each day which lasted only a few minutes. I had lots of time on my hands. I walked a lot and read. I was really afraid in the city.

The doctors and nurses at Beth Israel Hospital were fantastic. They treated me individually and made my appointments late on Monday and early on Friday, so I could coordinate my plane flights to be home every weekend. There was no discomfort in the treatments. Some of the patients complained of fatigue for an hour or so after treatment, but I felt nothing unusual. It was a 6-week program and during the last two weeks of treatment my skin began to burn. It became like a severe sunburn and I feared I may be scarred for life. The doctors assured me it would heal perfectly normally and showed me slides of patients from beginning to end, to confirm the theory. This was the most discomfort I had experienced thus far and sure enough, two weeks later my skin looked normal again.

One day I felt brave and asked my doctor to show me a slide of a patient who had a mastectomy. He came back with several colored slides. It was worse than I had ever imagined and knew for certain I would never question myself on having made the right decision

Back home for two weeks and then back to Beth Israel for the initial radiation implant. I flew up alone on Sunday and admitted myself to the hospital. Since I would be in isolation for 3 days, it would be useless for my husband to accompany me.

Monday morning I was put to sleep and they inserted the hollow tubes through my breast to make way for the radiation beads which would be threaded thru later when I was back in my room. I awoke with some discomfort but no violent pain. Pain shots were prescribed for me, but I refused them in lieu of an oral drug. I didn't want to be drugged to the point I could not remember.

On Thursday morning, the nurse came in and gave me 3 shots as I waited for the doctor who would remove the radiation beads. I expected the shots to numb me somewhat, but it seemed there was no change and the removal was a bit painful. The doctor told me I came through it like a champ and that I could go home. I called the airport for my reservation, got dressed and called a cab. At 10:45 am, I was on a plane bound for PA. At 12 noon my husband met me at the airport and by then I was a little woosey. But - I had made it - it was all over. The doctors had pronounced me a complete success. Prognosis - EXCELLENT!

I returned to my job the following Monday and back to a near normal life.

So you see there was an alternative to mastectomy - as early as 1977. I am a living example and thankful every day that God gave me the strength and courage to be my own person.

Betty lives in Belleville, PA.

A Friend in Need
Maria Kerstetter

I have been on the sidelines of cancer so far – one of the lucky ones. I share the stories of three people close to me who have battled cancer. One thing I've learned: to be a good friend – just 'be there.'

Story One...
My mother-in-law, Sharon Kerstetter, is a 27-year breast cancer survivor. The most important thing we have learned is that you need to have your family involved with you during the entire cancer process. The cancer patient may think she wants to save her family all the pain and heartache, but being able to share and be a part of the treatments, appointments, etc., helps everyone deal with the whole cancer process.

Our family has shared many tears, hugs, concerns, laughs and made lots of memories. Humor has also played a huge part in dealing with the nasty side of cancer. My mother-in-law has established the Boobless Wonder Club. Some may think 'how crude,' but when you are the one dealing with cancer 24/7, humor plays a big part in being able to cope with it. Sharon has played a huge part in helping a lot of women in Central PA to deal with the loss of one or both of their breasts, and to experience the hope that there are brighter days ahead while sharing some experiences from the past 27 years. Her most famous quote is that she is a winner either way; losing her battle with cancer, but spending eternity with her Lord.

Story Two...
A friend of mine found out she had breast cancer only a few months after losing her husband to Alzheimer's. She decided that humor will play a huge part in her recovery process, too. She came to church one week recently as a redhead and another week as a blond. She said, "If I get tired of being a blond, I will put my wig in the drawer and pick another color." She decided it would

196

be best for her to have her hair cut off all at one time than waking up every day with another hunk of hair missing. Humor is her way of dealing with the entire cancer process. Humor is her way of dealing with not having hair. It may not work for everybody, but it works for her.

Story Three…

My brother was 39 when he was diagnosed with Leukemia. We found out after it was too late for a bone marrow transplant. He was so weak that when he was diagnosed he was told if they had not found the cancer he would have been gone in two weeks.

Thankfully, the Lord gave us another year with him and the most important thing I learned was to be there for each other no matter what. I didn't even have to say a word if he was having a bad day. Just being there and holding his hand was enough; for both of us.

If you have someone going through cancer, don't worry about not having anything to say to him. Just being there is enough and means so much.

Maria lives in Blanchard, PA with her husband Troy and is employed at Centre County Christian Academy as the Administrative Secretary. Her husband is the Pastor at Faith Baptist Church in Blanchard, PA. They have three children, Chad 24, Renee 21, and Ashley 11. Her son is married to Sarah and her first grandchild, Baby K is due to arrive in September. She was born in Lewistown, PA and has lived in PA all of her life. She can be reached at mkerstetter@cccacademy.org.

List of Love
Lisa Klenoshek

If someone would have told me in the past that I would someday be sharing my personal breast cancer story, I would have laughed out loud! I never thought I would get cancer. In fact, I didn't think about cancer at all. I'm young, healthy, eat right, exercise, don't smoke and take vitamins. However, in the spring of 2009, my world took a hit.

Life was rolling along just fine until the phone call about my mammogram in April 2009. After an ultrasound and a very painful biopsy, I got the most shocking news ever. Breast Cancer! Actually, the words were, "It's cancer, my dear!" from my sweet radiologist, Dr. Gizienski. My schedule quickly changed and my calendar filled up. Two surgeries; a lumpectomy and total axillary dissection because of a couple cancer cells in a lymph node! Then it was more tests, port placement surgery, sixteen weeks of nasty, brutal chemotherapy and 35 radiation treatments. Finally, about 10 months later, I was finished with my treatment. Cancer free? That's what they tell me!

"Now go live your life. Forget about cancer." Donna from radiation said. Easier said than done!

Cancer has changed me. Sure, I look like the same old Lisa on the outside. But inside, I'm different. I would still consider myself a positive person. I think this helped me during my cancer battle. I'm thankful to be alive, but I'm scared of my future. I'm tired all the time. And something I struggle with is my own mortality, which is not a very positive way to live. Cancer took away my carefree life. For that, I'm angry. So I just try to trudge on, live life to the fullest and enjoy seeing my daughter, Zoey Rose, grow up.

Writing is one of my emotional releases. It was during my cancer battle I started writing. I did a daily journal on caringbridge.org. It started as a way to communicate to friends and family about my diagnosis, doctors' appointments and test results. But it also became therapeutic. My journal was a place to release my frustrations and anxiety, fears and concerns. One day my mom asked if I knew I had a "following"? That many people were reading my daily entries and waiting for the next one? Uh, no...I didn't know that! Turns out I did have a group of people reading my daily journal entries. And when I closed my journal in May 2010, after the Susan G. Komen Race for the Cure in Pittsburgh, it ended up being like a textbook! My site had 14,722 hits, 277 entries, 902 guestbook signings, and 50 pictures. It is now a great reference for me from that difficult time in my life.

Soon after I finished my journal, I wrote a children's book called Zoey's List of Love; A Sweet, Breast Cancer Survival Story. (Mirror Publishing, Oct. 2010) It's been a wonderful experience! I didn't know it at the time, but I have a mission. I want to help adults talk to kids about cancer. It's such a tough conversation. One of the low points during my cancer battle was when Zoey came to me with tears in her eyes and asked me, "Momma, are you going to die?" I was dumbfounded! I wasn't prepared. I hope that my book can help other parents talk to kids about this difficult process to wellness.

Zoey's List of Love is about a momma going through breast cancer and her little girl is scared but wants to help. Zoey writes lists along the way with her ideas on how to help Momma during her battle to wellness. This story just poured out of me and closely resembles many things that transpired in our house during treatment. And, Zoey is a list writer! She's a true inspiration to me in so many ways. Zoey knew something was wrong. She wanted to know what and she wanted to know how she could help, which I think helped her deal with the scary stuff happening at home. She wasn't used to seeing me on the couch with bandages after surgery. She didn't understand why I was so tired all of the time or why my hair fell out! The more we talked to her, the less afraid she was. Today, Zoey is a strong little girl who helped her Momma, me, battle cancer. I hope my book can help others.

Cancer has made me smarter.

I've learned that a sense of humor is always a good thing, even in the face of cancer. Like the time I was driving to pick up Zoey from kindergarten and realized, halfway there, that I didn't have anything on my bald head! I pulled the car over. I thought I must have a ball cap or something in the car to cover my head. Nope! Nothing! Except...Zoey's beloved blanket. Her Woobie. So I wrapped it around my bald dome like a turban and just smiled as her teacher helped Zoey into my back seat. A sense of humor is a must! Anyone who has gone wig shopping can attest to that, I'll bet!

I've learned that my head is nicely shaped. All my life, my Grandma June has told me that I have a nicely shaped head! In early August 2009, after my friend Tina shaved my head, I learned that she was right. And just as the last lock of hair was floating away from my head, I felt my first pang of sadness over losing my hair. Seconds later, my husband was reassuring me that I was beautiful and brave. I never looked back after that. He loves me for better or for worse, in sickness and in health, with hair and without. I'm a lucky girl.

Cancer has made me thankful.

1. I'm thankful that I got my mammogram. What if I had skipped it? I shudder to think about it.

2. I'm thankful for the thousands of women who participated in clinical trials before me so that I could receive the best treatments. I, too, participated in a trial during treatment.

3. I'm thankful for my husband and prince charming for being by my side every step of the way. And for my daughter, my inspiration for fighting and writing my first children's book. And for my parents! They did so much for us while I was going through treatment. And I'm thankful for all of my family and friends. Cancer taught me that I'm surrounded by amazing people in my life. I didn't realize how lucky I was in that department before my diagnosis on that Tuesday afternoon, May 12, 2009, when I first heard the words, "you have cancer."

I'm proud to be a survivor and part of a special sisterhood. I meet people all the time who notice a pink ribbon on me and stop to give me a hug. And share their story. And best of all, tell me how many years they have survived Breast Cancer.

My husband, Bill, and I are both very proud to be past our cancer battle. So proud, in fact, that one evening last summer we both got pink ribbon tattoos to symbolize our triumph over this dreaded disease!

Now I stay busy with raising Zoey, promoting my book to help other parents, and being a mentor for the American Cancer Society. There is a cure. We just have to find it. I truly believe that we will put an end to cancer sometime in this lifetime. I cannot wait until that day!

Poems by Lisa Klenoshek

Side Effects

The medicine cabinet was overflowing
My list of drugs growing and growing.
Compazine to keep the nausea at bay
Imitrex to make the headaches go away.
Feeling anxious? Take Zofran.
Can't sleep? Try Ativan.
And don't forget that weekly injection
Neulasta to help fight infection.
Infused with Anzemet, Benadryl, Cytoxane,
That nasty red devil, Adriamycin.
Vicodin was my saving grace
That pill put a smile on my face.
Side effects from side effects
Again something I didn't expect.
But the biggest thing I really hated…
All of those drugs made me constipated!

Precious Breath

Cancer can teach a crucial lesson
Each breath we take is precious.
Our time down here on Earth is undefined.
It's such an important message.

Live for the moment, don't look back.
The past cannot be undone.
Embrace your passions, take risks, help others,
Love with fearless abandon.

Eliminate stress; smile as often as possible.
Feel your heart go pitter-patter.
Focus on loved ones in need,
Make each precious breath matter.

Yes, cancer can bring to light one truth
That when we are summoned to the angels above
All that will have mattered on Earth
Is how much we were able to love.

OUCH!

Pulling pushing
Smashing smushing
Get closer
Turn right
Head back
Too tight!

Prodding kneading
Am I bleeding?
Hold still
Deep breath
So painful
Near death.

Ah, finished!
Pain diminished.
Time to go
My eyes wide
What did you say?
The other side!

Hat Party

No hair on my head?
"No worries" I said.
A hat party for me.
Many to choose from, thankfully.
Bucket hats in purple and peach
And denim and green within my reach.
A woven straw hat shields the sun
Or the red beret is really fun.
Sometimes a cowboy hat's my mood
Black leather or pink shows attitude.
Perhaps a handkerchief aqua or yellow
A silk flowered scarf on days I'm mellow.
At times a baseball cap will do
I choose from pink, white or blue.
For cold winter days a fuzzy knitted cap
It's easy to stay warm if you have earflaps.
So many head covers each day I pick
One to wear 'till my hair comes back thick!

It's Cancer, My Dear!

I'll never forget the dreaded call.
It wasn't the news I wanted to hear.
That sweet and caring doctor with her warm smiles
Delivered the words, "It's cancer, my dear."

I'll never forget the date….May twelfth,
Sitting at the kitchen table.
My doctor was telling me my future.
I was shaking, scared, and unstable.

Nine to twelve months of surgeries and treatments.
Life as I knew it changed.
In an instant I became a breast cancer patient,
My priorities rearranged.

I hung up the phone with pages of notes.
My husband grabbed me for a tight embrace.
I could think of only my 4 year old daughter.
I could only see her beautiful face.

And in a snap it was clear what I had to do.
Despite all concern and unease
I would fight! I would live! I would survive this news.
I would beat my breast cancer disease!

Chemo Brain
What did you say?
My mind was far away.
Chemo brain is to blame.

Where are my keys?
Are you talking to me?
Chemo brain is to blame.

Did I feed the cat?
Oops. Forgot about that.
Chemo brain is to blame.

So much fog in my head.
I'm the living dead.
Chemo brain is to blame.

When will clarity return?
For a clear thought I yearn.
Before chemo brain strikes again!

Lisa, a 2 Year Triple Negative B.C. Survivor, was born in western Pennsylvania, but raised in Port Clinton, Ohio. She's a business graduate of Miami University in Oxford, Ohio and currently resides in Cranberry Township near Pittsburgh, Pennsylvania, where she loves being a stay-at-home mom. When she's not writing, Lisa is baking something yummy or practicing the piano! She lives with her husband, Bill, and their daughter, Zoey Rose. Visit Lisa's website at www.LisaKBooks.com.

Knowledge is Power
Diane Kline

I first learned I had breast cancer in January 2000. What a way to start a new millennium. Being the factual analytical person that finance people usually are, we have this built in need to know.

I then went to work fighting my fears with knowledge. I researched every word on my pathology report on the internet, to early hours in the morning. I had no trouble sleeping that night because I was exhausted. I also went to bed with a plan in my head. I said to myself, "Okay, let's take care of this and move on."

Knowledge is power and the unknown creates fear, the more you learn about your condition the more likely you will be to make educated choices that are right for you.

Diane Kline lives in Lewistown, PA with her husband Danny Kline and her two labs Zeke and Lexi Ann. She works at the Lewistown Hospital in the Finance Department and can be reached by e-mail at dkline@lewistownhospital.org.

Dear Cancer...
Diana Klunk

Unfortunately most of us have had cancer touch our lives…some of us have had cancer ourselves, or a spouse has had cancer, or a parent, a sibling, another relative or, God forbid, a child. Or you may have helped a friend, or a neighbor or a co-worker who has battled this disease in one form or another. I personally have had my life touched in many ways. I am a breast cancer survivor, the spouse of a colon cancer survivor, the sister of a melanoma survivor, the daughter in law of a prostate cancer survivor and sister in law of a testicular cancer survivor, my father died of lung cancer two and a half years ago, and my mother is currently undergoing chemo for colon cancer. Even in the face of all of this I want to thank cancer for its impact on my life.

It all started on Tuesday, December 26, 2006. I had my annual mammogram, and the tech told me we needed to take more views because of micro calcifications in my right breast. I had a very strong gut feeling right then and there that I had cancer – call it intuition, or whatever – and I was scheduled for a stereotactic biopsy on Friday. In the meantime I went to see my surgeon, who performed a core needle biopsy to test the tissue for cancer. On Friday December 28 at 9 AM the doctor called to confirm my fears…*I had breast cancer at age 47.*

Contrary to popular belief, you do not become a cancer survivor after your treatment has ended…you become a survivor as soon as you are diagnosed. One second after you hear those 3 dreadful words – *you have cancer* – you have survived with cancer for 1 second, and thus you become a survivor.

So now it was time to make some decisions. LOTS of doctor appointments and medical tests – will I need surgery, chemo, radiation? One of the decisions I needed to make was if I wanted to try to save my breasts….and, I decided not to try to save mine. In addition to the cancer that was in my right breast the MRI detected some suspicious areas in the left breast, and I opted for a double mastectomy with immediate TRAM flap reconstruction, which means they took my abdominal fat and muscles and moved them up through my ribcage to form new breasts with my own body tissue. It was a long 9 ½ hour surgery, performed at Hanover Hospital on February 6, 2007, and I did remarkably well. Also during this time we found out that my Dad was diagnosed with lung cancer. While I was preparing to fight for my life through continued treatment, he opted not to have any treatment.

March 20, 2007 was my first of eight rounds of dose-dense chemotherapy, and it was time to hit this head on with everything that I had. I went every two weeks to receive the toxic drugs into my body that would hopefully kill off any errant cancer cells that may have escaped. Although my 5.1 cm tumor, which was the size of a lime, was removed when I had the bilateral mastectomy, I also had two positive lymph nodes out of the 19 that were removed. That meant that the cancer had spread outside of the breast and needed to be treated very aggressively. I was very fortunate during chemo and did not experience too many bad side effects, but I did lose my hair after 14 days.

Twenty weeks later, after I had finished my chemo, I started 32 radiation treatments, which I also tolerated fairly well. In September I had both ovaries and fallopian tubes removed as an extra precaution, and in October, after nine months off, I returned to my position as an accounting associate.

Then, on December 22, 2007, my husband was diagnosed with colorectal cancer. He did not have any symptoms of any kind...he simply had a screening colonoscopy performed because he turned 50 that May and our daughter and I insisted that he get this done. We were as totally unprepared for his diagnosis as we were for mine, but once again we found ourselves visiting doctors and making decisions on what the next step should be.

In early January 2008 my husband had 12" of his colon removed and resectioned. Fortunately his cancer was an early stage, was completely contained in the polyp that was removed during his colonoscopy, and we were told he would not need any further treatment. Unfortunately he had some complications from the original surgery and 16 days later he had to return to the hospital for another surgery. This was a setback but he was able to return to work 9 weeks later and thankfully remains cancer free today.

At this point, you are probably wondering how I could possibly want to say "Thank You" to cancer. There are many reasons for me to say thank you. So please let me share with you my thank you letter to cancer:

Dear Cancer,

I wanted to take this opportunity to thank you for the impact you have made on my life. I do not thank you for the changes and scars my body has experienced as a result of you, the "chemo brain" that is a result of aggressive chemotherapy, or the pain and fears and tears you inflicted on my family and friends. However, I do want to thank you for so many things…for making me realize that just because a job pays well, that is not reason enough to keep doing it if your mind and heart are not in to it, that if you follow your dreams you will never regret it and that if you have an opportunity to reach out and help someone else by all means do it. I was not satisfied in my accounting career but had no idea what I wanted to do instead and you changed all of that.

From the beginning, within days after I was diagnosed, God planted the seed for me to do something more meaningful with my life. Knowing that I would need a wig if I had chemo, I visited a boutique to see what my options were. Although the store itself was lovely, I was not anxious to have to visit such a place. To add insult to injury I was not greeted when I entered the store nor acknowledged at all until I approached the girl behind the desk to inquire about a wig. She pointed to a room in the back and told me to help myself…the wig person was not in. I tried on a few wigs (I think I got them on right!) and left feeling so much worse than when I went in. I later learned about products that were right there in front of me that would have made my life and my recovery a whole lot easier, had I known about them, but no one bothered to talk to me or ask me any questions about what my diagnosis was or what my treatment plan was. I went home and told my husband that I wanted to open a similar type of boutique to help women going through the same experiences as me, only I wanted to treat them with dignity, respect and compassion as soon as they walked through the door. And so the concept for LifeChanges was born….

All during my treatment and recovery and my husband's experience with you I just could not make this idea go away – God speaks in many ways. If anything, it continued to grow. In early 2008, I started to seriously research making this dream a reality. After a trip to Albuquerque to a trade show and convention I knew I was ready to take the plunge. I approached Hanover Hospital with my idea, and they were very supportive from the start. They offered me open space they had available to lease for my location, and I was on my way. I received great guidance and support from two women who own a beautiful boutique and allowed me to visit them and shadow them. On October 1, 2008, two months after you took my Dad from me, cancer, LifeChanges Boutique, a health and healing boutique for women living with cancer, opened.

At **LifeChanges**, our mission is to provide the products, services and support that women with cancer need in a warm, compassionate environment. We offer a wig salon, head coverings and hats, mastectomy bras, fittings and prostheses, mastectomy swimsuits and compression hosiery and garments. In addition we carry t-shirts including those I have shared with you today, along with hand crafted jewelry, Lindsay Phillips shoes, Bauble LuLu beads and a variety of other products – something for everyone, not just for cancer survivors. We also offer a shoulder to cry on and the opportunity to sit down and speak to someone who's "been there". I am involved in fundraising and support of the American Cancer Society through Relay For Life, and also **The Pink Out** Women's Cancer Fund and Pink Ribbon Challenge as a committee member for these events. We also offer the ACS's "Look Good Feel Better" program every third Monday, and I co-facilitate the Hanover Area Breast Cancer Support Group, also on the third Monday of the month.

And so, cancer, I would like to tell you that I have been blessed in many ways, and owe some of those blessings to you. However, I also want you to know that I will do everything within my power to help rid you from our bodies and our lives. I can not only imagine a world without cancer but hope to see that become a reality in my lifetime, so my grandchildren do not have to know any more about you then they already do, and so that others do not have to go through the heartbreak of hearing those three words, "you have cancer".

I have been led by God to dedicate the remainder of my professional life to serving others, and helping them through what might just be the worst time of their life. If I can do one thing to help, offer one word of advice, or put a smile on a face that has not smiled for a while, then it was worth going through the cancer experience myself. And, I AM a survivor!

Diana is a lifelong resident of Hanover, PA. She is married to Ken, has two children and four grandchildren. She is the president of LifeChanges Boutique, Inc in Hanover and is also a member of the Pink Out Committee, Pink Ribbon Challenge Golf Tournament Committee, is active in local American Cancer Society activities and also Main Street Hanover and the Hanover Chamber Of Commerce.

We Are Not Riding Alone
Vicki Kovatto

My story started while I was preparing for a breast reduction surgery. For many years, I had back pain from my breast and I felt at this point in my life, I was ready to reduce the pain (and the pain causers!). I had the biggest boobs in the history of mankind! So when I found out that I was actually getting rid of them altogether rather than just have them reduced, I thought.... Wow, this is one way to lose weight. One of my friends who was not full-figured asked me if I would donate them to her....you know, like donating a kidney. Heck, I had enough boobs to outfit 5 women!

During the testing that you go through in preparation for the surgery, a mammogram showed there was something suspicious. I always had regular mammograms, which often showed cysts, but I never expected the diagnosis that followed.

After an extremely painful lumpectomy (surgery from hell), on December 8, 2003, I was diagnosed with Lobular Neoplasia, which is a pre-cancer that mirrors itself, and is a marker for cancer in women. I had a bi-lateral mastectomy on March 10, 2004, and had implants placed in my breasts. Just this past January 10, 2011, I had the implants removed due to scar tissue and tightness in my chest. I did not require chemo or radiation. I still have my lymph nodes. I have not had any issues since.

Even though this was a serious situation, I try to find humor in everything and I am quick to smile and laugh. Throughout the situation, I tried to poke fun at myself, maybe doing it for the children's sake as much as my own.

My sister, Betty "Jo" Rivera (her story is also in this book) was diagnosed with Invasive Ductal Carcinoma, stage 3 in 2006. She had her right breast removed. She suffered through over six months of chemo and radiation. She was also given the new drug, Herceptin (via a port) for a full year. Her lymph nodes were removed from her right side. She had quite a bad time of it. In her opinion, the Herceptin saved her life. She calls it her "miracle drug". She is one of a group of five breast cancer survivors. Out of the five girls, all nurses, two have since had their cancer return and have passed away. My sister, so far is cancer free.

My sister is married but never had children. I am divorced and have two adult children. My sister had a gene screening done to make sure that we didn't have the cancer gene in our family, and we do not. Regardless, I am fearful for both of my children. My mother and father (while in their 70's when they passed) both had cancer. My sister, who works as an RN at St. Joseph's in Reading, PA, truly believes we are eating, drinking and breathing cancer. Two of my co-workers just recently survived breast cancer as well. It does seem to be all around us.

Even though there is a lot of cancer around us, I firmly believe that we cannot dwell on it, but we must choose to live, really live each day. As I said, I like to have fun, in spite of the things in life that can get us down from time to time. Not too long ago, we had a Staff Appreciation Luncheon. I thought I would shake things up a bit so I wore my sister's wig that she had from her chemo and I took one of my pre-surgery bras and stuffed it with socks. (After the surgery and the removal of my implants, well, there isn't as much "up top" as there used to be.) I now use socks for my ta-tas, and I just want you to know…it takes three pair!!!

Tammy asked me to respond to how I view life. How do I view life? Holy cow, where do I begin? Just to wake up every morning, knowing that I am going to take care of my two dogs that day…and that both my children are healthy is like touching God's hand. I can't describe it. Just the other day my sister Jo told me her Doctors declared her "cured". Can you imagine that? My sister is cured. We are so rich, so, so rich. I love that feeling.

What would I say to a newly diagnosed person to encourage or inspire them? Well, it's like falling off a horse. You pick yourself up, brush off the tumbleweed, hop back on and finish the ride. You can't feel sorry for yourself because there is always someone else in worse shape. ***You can do this***. And most importantly, have faith. You are not finishing that ride alone.

Life is too short not to have fun! Take each day, embrace your life and have fun!

Vicki Kovatto
Assisted by Tammy Miller

(Family story of Vicki Kovatto, Jo Rivera, Miguel Rivera, Alexis Pino, and Michael Pino)

Vicki is 60 years old and has a great job at Penn State University. She has two wonderful adult children (Alexis and Michael Pino – their stories are also in this book) and two wonderful dogs. She has a multitude of "close" friends. She says she has no chest, and her tummy area looks like Mrs. Doubtfire. She loves quilting, and crocheting, and she takes pride in being the best of the best when it comes to cooking and baking.

Moving Forward
Marge Kresge

It was October 2006 and I knew it was time for my yearly mammogram. I always made sure to schedule it for the month of October because it was Breast Cancer awareness month and that would help me remember to make the appointment. I had routine mammograms for many years so I knew what to expect, but this time it was different.

The routine was the same, I went in, got the exam, waited for the films to be read and left. The difference this time was that I got a call a couple of days later saying they needed more films. I had never had this happen before and I was very frightened. I shared my concerns with my daughters and husband when I told them I had to go for more tests.

After the additional films were done I had to wait for the doctor. I was very nervous at this point and not sure of what was going on. The radiologist walked into the room and said, "Marge we saw some things on the films and you need to see an Oncologist".

I was very frightened and did not know what to expect. The first doctor I saw I did not like at all and I didn't go back. I had decided that this was very serious and I needed someone I could trust and would take the time to answer my questions. Fortunately, the second doctor I went to was wonderful. He had a great bedside manner and was highly recommended by anyone I spoke with about what was happening. One thing that he did that I really liked was he started taping everything we talked about for me to take home and listen to. He wanted to make sure I had the information in case I got home and couldn't remember what he said.

Breast cancer wasn't really talked about, I was numb and shocked going through everything that was happening. It took my sister in law sitting me down and shaking some sense into me for me to realize I had it. I was stage zero, and in my mind that means you don't have it, "zero" means nothing, right? It took my sister in law really telling me "listen you have breast cancer" for it to sink in.

The hardest part for me was that my oldest daughter was pregnant, and my youngest daughter was planning her wedding – I just didn't have time to have cancer!

I had a battery of surgeries starting with a lumpectomy in December of 2006, and then they did another lumpectomy in February 2007. After that surgery the doctor called me and said that I didn't have a choice, I needed the mastectomy. It was the first time I didn't have a choice, I knew it was best if he was telling me it was best.

My first grand daughter was born in March – a beautiful bright spot in all of the turmoil.

Following the mastectomy I had the reconstruction, which was very a difficult procedure. After the reconstruction I got an infection and a hernia and the whole episode turned out to be a bad situation. It was a total of four surgeries within one year and I could have done without the whole experience. At first I was in total shock and withdrawn. I tried to keep everything inside and pay attention to their needs, but it was difficult to function some days as there was so much going on in my head.

I was going about my day like nothing was happening, not knowing what was going on inside my body. With everything going on with my daughters, there wasn't time for a pity party, and there wasn't a lot of time to really think about what was happening, which was probably a very good thing.

Slowly but surely I started to talk with people about what was happening in my life (and my body!), and I started to feel better about the whole process. I believe this is when I started to heal mentally. Since I had my surgery about three hours from where I live, I didn't feel a real connection to the women in my home area. I think this disconnect slowed the mental healing process.

I am very thankful for my family and I leaned heavily on them. I had a lot of positive help from my family and friends. A positive circle around you can help you deal with a lot more than you think you can. I could not have done it without them. I don't think there is ever a "right time" for something like this, but if there ever was in my life, this was the time. With all of the energy and excitement about the birth of my grand daughter and my daughter's wedding, my mind was focused in different directions.

My daughter reminded me of the Rascal Flatts song, "Stand". The theme of the song is to overcome obstacles in your life by standing in "victory" when things are tough. Some of the lyrics are, *You get mad, you get strong, wipe your hands, shake it off, then you stand, yeah, then you stand.* I kept that song with me during the year to help me get through my surgeries and infections. It is kind of my theme song.

At Penn State we have a woman's basketball game called the Pink Zone that is dedicated to breast cancer. Because of some of the people involved, it has become more of a celebration of life. I hesitated to attend, but I finally gave in and was very glad I did. At the event I started to talk to people and started to realize that I was not alone, that there were many women going through this challenge and we all have a different story.

My words to encourage others would be that it's going to be a roller coaster ride – you are going to have ups and downs throughout your journey. Listen to your doctors, take what you can from them, and hang in there. It is going to be a ride, be informed, make your decisions and stick with them. Make your decisions only after you digest everything.

I am concerned about my daughter and I certainly do not want them to go through what I endured. I pray there is a cure before too long and that my daughter and grand daughters will not have to go through this pain and challenge.

What I would want other women to know is to educate yourself. After I had my reconstruction I wasn't aware of the infection risks. I had home health care coming in to help take care of me during my recovery. It was nice because I was able to be in my own home, but it was my only option since I had the surgery at a hospital three hours away.

Tammy asked me to think about anything humorous that may have happened during this time. I can't recall very much, but the one day Dr. M "zoomed" into the room, just before my surgery and wrote all over my body with a purple marker. For some reason, this struck me as funny. I felt like I was a piece of art work.

I think the funniest thing that happened to me during my experience was while I was recovering, I went in for a follow up with my doctor and he said to me, with a straight face, "I am surprised you don't have a nipple tattooed on here yet". It shocked me that he was making a joke with everything I was going through but it was nice to lighten the mood, and it made me smile. He was very relaxed and that helped me relax. I believed in my doctor, I trusted this man, and he was the man who saved my life.

Marge Kresge
As written by Lacey Earnest

Marge lives in Bellefonte, Pa with her husband Dave. She had two daughters both happily married, 2 beautiful granddaughters, and 1 handsome grandson. She works full time, and enjoys spending time with her family.

How I Cheated on My Hairdresser
Rae Lanzendorfer

This is the story of why, where, with whom and how I cheated on my hairdresser. But let me start at the beginning. I have for many years gone to a wonderful woman and hairdresser. Never any issues with her work, as a matter of fact, I felt sorry for her that she had to find a way to make my hair look good.

Last year, I was given some devastating news that I had breast cancer. I was ready for the fight. Chemotherapy, surgery and radiation would be the soldiers in my battle. I would be the general who would have to put up with what their effects would be. What does this have to do with my hairdresser? Well, the day finally came when enough of my hair had fallen out that I decided to shave it off. They say that a woman will know when to go bald and I had reached that day. My husband offered, but I felt that it would be too traumatic for him and me. I decided that my hairdresser would do the deed. So, on my way home from work, I stopped in at her salon. This was the first she had heard of my diagnosis and was willing to help me in my battle. She stopped at the point where my hair looked like a man's buzz cut. The reflection in the mirror screamed "you look like your brother" so I told her to shave it all off. She would not take my money, but left me with her words of encouragement. I felt had finally crossed the "losing my hair" hurtle. I sent her a thank you card letting her know what she had done for me.

Fast forward to the next year, chemos over, surgery's done and radiation complete and for good measure throw in a hysterectomy. My hair came back as the straight, salt and pepper hair I had before. I went back to her in the fall to have her style it, as soon as I had enough hair to stop wearing a wig, which wasn't much. My chemo friends who had lost their hair had much longer hair than I did at this point. My hair grew in but was not growing fast enough to be the style I wanted. I felt destined to have very short ugly unruly hair

One day in March, I went shopping with my sister-in-law. I started to pity myself, because I just could not look in a store mirror without welling up in tears. I asked her if we could stop at a local salon that was not too far from where we were to ask for suggestions about what to do with my hair. They were having a special that day, a shampoo and style. My sister-in-law said that she wanted to get this for me for my birthday, which was only a few short weeks away. I agreed and when the young woman stylist was done with my hair, I felt as if a part of my old self had returned. Upon checking out, I was told that if I booked again in 6 weeks I could get the same special. Feeling the way that I did about my hair at that moment, I scheduled an appointment.

Six weeks passed and my appointment day had arrived. Although my hair had not grown much, I wanted to feel as I did after my first appointment. Little did I know that I was in for a real treat. My hair was to be styled by a young gay man, who tried out for a reality show called, Shear Genius. I have never had someone spend so much time on my hair; then again I had never paid so much to have my hair cut. He did most of the talking, which I enjoyed, because his conversation was more interesting than mine, so I continued to ask him question. Besides a new style he gave me some low-lights and then took me over to the makeup counter to have my face made up.

I walked out of the salon again feeling great, but I knew that I would never see him again, even though the experience was priceless. I love my hairdresser; she gives me routine, which is also a comforting feeling that is also priceless. Besides, she was there for me at the beginning of my breast cancer journey.

So on my way home from work, I stopped in to make an appointment with my hairdresser and told her that "I cheated on you" and then I told tell her the story. She laughed and said 'your hair really looks good' and then proceeded to ask me what I would like done and when did I want to come in. I felt home again and it felt good.

My Hairdresser: Janna, A Cut Above the Rest, Park Hill, PA

Crossing Paths

They say that there are reasons that people's paths cross in life. I did not know her well, but do we really need to know everything about someone to complete a relationship. She came into my life a year and a half ago though a mutual friend, Pat, when I had a big decision to make about whether to have a bilateral mastectomy. She imparted her experience and wisdom to me at a time when decisions were not so easy for me and I was doing through chemotherapy. We talked on the phone and corresponded through e-mails. I could not have asked for a kinder person to help me make a decision that I am happy with to this day

We said through e-mails that one day we would meet. So, in July when I decided to visit the local area to see my brother and my friend, Pat, the decision was an easy one. I would visit her. Not having her home phone number, I called Pat to see if she could get it for me. Dialing from my brother's home, she answered the phone and told me to come over to visit. Arriving at her home, I felt calmed by the surroundings and serene in her presence. You always wonder about a person's physical appearance when you have never met them. I was not surprised, she was beautiful, not only on the outside, but she radiated beauty from the inside.

We greeted each other with a hug and went to sit on her porch. She graciously offered me something to drink and then told me that she never picks up the phone showing numbers she did not know, but this time she did. I thanked her for that decision. We talked about our disease, breast cancer, our homes, our work, and Pat. The hours that we spent together were so relaxing. She made it that way. She said that maybe we would be able to see each other again, but I knew that the distance between where we both lived along with the battle she was waging again with cancer would not make that easy. We hugged and I left happy, knowing that I finally got to meet her and thinking how lucky her family and friends are.

Now it is October and today, I got the call from Pat that she had passed. I felt sad and numb, but compelled to tell the story of what she had done for me. Small events in life often go unrecognized by others. They remain a memory for only those who experience them. So, this is the story of my crossing paths with Karen Dwyer-Jones and the impression she made and left in my life.

Pearls of Wisdom

This story is about two women who have endured and conquered obstacles in their personal lives imparting wisdom to each other along the way. I will not go into the history of their friendship or the heartaches they both have endured, but will tell of the two days in December where they spent quality time together at a spa in Berkeley Springs West Virginia. Their names are Pat and Rae.

They wanted to get together, but had to find a place between where they both lived since Pat had moved away from the area several years earlier. Over the years since her move, they have kept in touch and remained as I like to say "friends of the mind", as they both seemed to have the uncanny ability to know when each other needed to speak to the other and the phone would ring.

Plans were made before Thanksgiving to meet in Berkeley Springs to do a spa day at the mineral baths along with a massage. Reservations were made at a hotel and the spa, but there was one problem that was putting a cloud over the entire planned retreat something Pat did not know. Rae was having problems with her breast and had received a call from her gynecologist's office to make an appointment with a surgeon. She made her appointment for five days after the retreat, but there was one problem, when to tell Pat, before to give her a heads up or let her know in Berkeley Springs. Rae thought, ruin it before or during. Her final decision was made; discuss the situation face to face in West Virginia, not over the phone.

Pat arrived at the hotel first with Rae arriving an hour later. They embraced, laughed and talked. At this point Rae decided to get the breast conversation over with. Pat looked stunned when Rae explained the condition of her breast. So, only a visual would do. They went into the bathroom and Rae"de-braed". Pat's first words were "God, they're huge." Laughter filled the bathroom, but there was a seriousness that suddenly stopped the laughter. Pat had unfortunately had to deal with a breast cancer diagnosis last year. It was decided that the "breast conversation" was over and they would have a good time as planned, so, off they went to find good food eventually ending up at an authentic Mexican restaurant and in all places, West Virginia. Then it was back to the hotel for wine, good conversation and sleep.

The next day was the scheduled mineral bath and massage. The bath was excellent and the massage hit the spot after the bath. They walked the town looking at the quaint shops and, of course, in search of food. There was a café that looked interesting with a unique atmosphere and an excellent menu. So, the decision was made and good food was consumed with pleasure. Next on the list was a visit to check out the County Inn and sit at the bar. After a beer, it was then decided that there was the need for one last mineral bath at the roman bath house. So off they went to partake again in the healing waters of Berkeley Springs. Feeling tired after the very hot bath, it was back to the hotel for a siesta before consuming more food and wine.

At the hotel, they enjoyed some wine, conversation and television. On a news program they were watching, there was a segment on Michele Obama. Pat mentioned the pearls that Michele frequently wears. Rae said that she bought a set of pearls on her thirtieth wedding anniversary, a long strand, kind of like the type won by Carrie in Sex in the City. The conversation moved onto other topics. It was decided to get ready for dinner at the Inn, which turned out to be the only disappointment of their retreat.

The next day was sad but at the same time joyful for the time that they had spent together. There is a quote that states "parting is such sweet sorrow"; on this day truer words were never spoken. They discussed a future retreat, but both understood that this would all depend on Rae's diagnosis.

It is now March and Rae has been diagnosed in December with Inflammatory breast cancer and is currently going through chemo and waiting for surgery. Pat has been more than a concerned friend. She has been a source of comfort and encouragement during the past months for Rae. So, for all of the wisdom that they have imparted to each other and as a symbol of their friendship, Rae has gifted her "strand of pearls" to Pat for her to keep and wear during the next year of Rae's cancer journey. This gift is also given with the hope that when this journey is over, they will be able to go on their second annual retreat.

This story was written for my Sister-friend, Pat,

Love, Rae

Rae lives in Strongstown, PA, with her husband of 36 years, Mark. She has an adult son and daughter, two grandsons and one granddaughter on the way. She has worked for Cambria County for almost 24 years and currently is the County Fiscal Officer with Drug and Alcohol. She can be reached at mdorfer@comcast.net

Cupcakes
Honey Leas

When my dear friend, Bonita, was going through her cancer two years ago, she was going through all the surgery etc., of course and I felt helpless and wanted to make things better. That's me - I try to fix things.

Anyway, she was dreading the 5 days a week for 6 weeks of radiation so I came up with the theme----"HOPE YOUR RADIATION JOURNEY IS A PIECE OF CAKE". Each week when she finished there was a cupcake of some kind, (first the floral, and then anything that I could find with a cupcake on it, a photo holder, candle container, pin cushion, etc.) Since cupcakes were not as popular a couple of years ago I ran out of ideas before the last appointment and ended up with a sailboat photo holder so the new message was, "Hope it is smooth sailing from now on". Bonita said the little gifts did help relieve the tension.

I am also a scrap booker so naturally I scrapbooked her cancer journey. The photos were of her team of doctors, the flowers and plants she received, even the vase full of daffodils for daffodil days. The tons of emails went in, a few of the best get well cards, the nurses, a photo of the new (then) breast cancer rose- which is a beautiful pink, and there is some stuff available to buy.

On one of her follow up appointments Bonita took her book in to show the surgeon. Dr. Smith loved it and wanted one for her office--so I made her a copy of Bonita's. It now holds a place of honor at the desk. Many other patients have sent letters, photos, etc. to add to her book.

Bonita and I both knit chemo caps for the local hospital, and enjoy the opportunity to help others with their journey.

In writing this I realized that I used what skills I had to try to make the journey a little easier for Bonita, and I think that is the best advice I can give.

Honey Leas and Bonita Hix live in southern CA. Now that they are both retired from teaching, they have a lot more time for all of their other interests: quilting, scrapbooking, stamping, traveling, volunteering, playing with their 2 cats (Patches & Buttons),etc. They can be reached at HoneyBonitaSew@aol.com

Beautiful Bernadette - A Thank You Letter
Alison LaVasseur

There are certain critical elements in our lives that create the proverbial foundation of which we truly are, whose lives we touch, and what we eventually become, and you Bernadette were the epitome of these fundamental values.

You were the warm loving arms of a mother who tucked your children in at night with butterfly kisses, the quintessential partner and loving wife to your husband, the soulful artist that captured every precious moment on film in hopes of preserving that infinite second that gave you unwavering happiness and joy. You were a daughter, a sister, a sister-in-law and friend, and above all else you were loved.

Bernadette you refused to let your illness destroy your life and home because you were strong in your beliefs, and your very life was defined by your home. After all, a home is a creation or culmination of family coming together and creating an invisible structure that calls to you as soon as you walk out the door. Home is the heartbeat that keeps us grounded because the idea of home is the single place that every person tries to get back to, no matter where their journey in life brings them. Home to YOU was invaluable.

In many ways you went to war when this cancer threatened and then invaded the very place that you fought so hard to create. You fought not only for yourself, but for that foundation you built slowly over time: a physical space built brick by brick, a mystical space built memory by memory, with the main component that is love. Love for each other, love for life, and the reason why no matter how far we travel, how successful we become, our ultimate goal is to come back home. Home is where your heart is. And no one understood that better than you.

You marched valiantly into war against this insidious disease. Initially humor was your weapon of choice. You made sure that when faced with the most heartbreaking moments, you had the knack to infuse laughter with tears. No one could have predicted that when we became lost in the basement of the hospital after you received a radioactive dye, consequently setting off the radiation detectors whereby hospital security tracked us down to secure the area, would lead to one of the funnier moments in an otherwise devastating journey. No one could have predicted the many hours spent "tailgating" while we waited long hours to see the doctors. We packed gourmet breakfast, lunch and dinners. The only thing missing was the Cosmos! At times we laughed so much that we would be asked to "quiet down" during chemo sessions because we were laughing too loud. No one could have predicted the poor target team member who commented on your beautiful hair, and you crying, subsequently sending the target team member home for the day!

During our long days and sometimes nights at the hospital, we spoke intimately about all the times in your life that were so incredulous. We talked about you writing a book. A book that would be about laughter and joy in the worst of times. We talked about you never giving up the fight, and how you so desperately wanted to be there for your daughter's proms, graduations and weddings. No one could have predicted that the battle was just beginning!

As the days became more difficult, and the cancer more aggressive, your battle became a full-blown war. The laughter became less and less, and during one of those sad days you asked me a particularly difficult question. You asked, "Why would this be my fate?" If my dad is watching over me, why would he allow this to happen to me?"

And I told you the following. Your dad is not allowing this to happen to you. Your dad left you the most precious gift anyone could receive. He left you his ESSENCE. His essence is the very foundation of who you are, how you live your life, how you created your HOME, and who you aspire to be. Your choices in how you live your life are based on those very same principles that he instilled in you. His essence is You! It was a bit of a light bulb moment for both us.

And to my beautiful sweet nieces, I tell you this, "Your mother's essence has been with you since the day you were born, and will always be a shining light deep within you. When you smile, she smiles, when you laugh, she laughs, and when you cry, her Essence will give you the strength and courage to laugh even in the toughest moments of your lives. Just like the gift your grandfather left to your mom."

What's important today is to realize that during those extremely difficult times in your life, draw on the essence of those loved and lost. That Essence creates a permanent footprint no matter where home is, which forever ties us to together. It is the very foundation of your lives. It won't heal the grief you feel because "Grief is by its nature unmanageable. The most we can do is respect its might and then ride it like a wave until it dumps us back on the shore." The ocean's rolling waters may wash away footprints left behind, but cannot by its very nature erase the beauty and essence of your soul.

From this day on, our Lives and our Home will forever be the foundation of our family because Bernadette, you are the very core of what makes a HOUSE A HOME, and although there are few words to articulate my extreme gratitude for having been a part of your life, I Thank You for leaving me your Essence. It is a gift that I shall cherish for the rest of my life.
Welcome Home!

Forever A Part of My Heart and Home - With All My Love
Alison

Alison is charmed in love and in life. She is fortunate enough to live in a small arts and crafts community in Rose Valley, Pennsylvania, with her husband Mike of 30 years. They have a beautiful 22 year old daughter Ariel (who has been forced to explain that her parents did not name her after a Disney character - The Little Mermaid was released 6 mos. after her birth), who recently graduated from Widener University, did not boomerang back home, and secured a full-time position in her field. When she is not working as a Paralegal/Marketing Assistant, she utilizes her spare time getting the word out that "Laughter Truly Is The Best Medicine."

A Sprinkle of FUN from Tammy...

"Each your carrot cake, Sweetie, yes, carrots are a vegetable!!"
--Tammy

Give Me a Head with Hair...
Gloria Libkin

It is amazing how or what encourages our feelings. Confidence comes from our families, our successes and our adventures. Our self-esteem is also created by how we feel about our looks. I was lucky in one way; I had great hair.

My hair was my best feature. It was light blond at a time when blond was in. Dumb blond jokes could go right over my head because I knew I was smart. And I was a teenager in the era of the Beach Boys with beach party girls and their long straight, blond hair. Peter, Paul and Mary sang at civil rights demonstrations. Mary's straight blond hair swung just like mine when she sang. I loved that friends envied my hair. They used peroxide and giant curlers to get the look that came naturally to me. Some even went so far as to iron their hair. I was horrified at the image of hair being pressed on an ironing board.

My hair remained a source of pride well into my 50's. It stayed light blond, only adding strawberry highlights and a bit of white around the temples.

At 56, my life changed. I needed to undergo chemotherapy for breast cancer. I lost my hair; gone was my best feature; gone was my blond hair framing my round face. Now here's the shocker. I looked just fine bald. I never thought I'd be OK without my blond hair, but I kind of liked the image change.

I grew personally through this experience, and eventually so did my hair. I found that my identity was not so tied to my hair any more. What freedom, although every once in a while, I catch myself wanting to explain to someone that my hair was light blond.

Gloria Libkin
As written by Kathy Salloum
Gloria retired in 2010 after many years as a school counselor. She lives in State College with her husband, Cary, and their two dogs. Her daughter Miranda, lives in Philadelphia. She wishes everyone sparkling light and time to breathe.

Loving the "Good"
Kelly Livergood

I received my phone call with "the news" at work on 3/3/10. I immediately called my husband and told him that now was his chance to leave, that I was broken. He told me – I love you and we're in this together. He hung up and came right to my office. We hugged and cried, then told my coworkers and boss. I stayed at work to finish out the day and my husband went home to begin the task of calling family.

One thing I have learned that has really helped me cope is that with every piece of bad news-there is always something good. My husband, Steve worked out of town for 15 years and was only home on weekends. He was just newly laid off. That was the bad news. The good - he was home when I needed him most. The bad - I was diagnosed with Stage IIA breast cancer—the good - I took out a Cancer policy thru my employer the year before my diagnosis!

We have two sons and it was not easy telling them. They are both very loving, caring and great sons. The hardest person to tell, though, was my youngest brother. He lost his first-born son at the young age of 10 to cancer in 2003. My nephew, Dylan was 8 when he was diagnosed with osteosarcoma. He battled this dreadful disease for 2 years and we watched him slowly die. My husband called him, as I just wasn't up to that.

We have been actively involved in the Relay for Life with the American Cancer Society for a number of years - beginning when Dylan was first diagnosed. At our relay in 2010, my family all came for support. When it came time for the Survivors Lap - words can't express how emotional I was. It was totally overwhelming to see my brother clap for me - but at the same time wishing that his son was also walking that lap! The bad - the guilt I am personally dealing with for beating this and why not Dylan – the good - that it was me with cancer and not my sons, not my husband, not my elderly mother, not my sister, not my brothers and most of all not either of my other little nephews.

232

The good - I have learned a lot and realized how much Dylan went through, although I thought I had an idea - but found out I didn't have a clue! Dylan is my hero and will always be. He was a child and never got to experience his first date, kiss, prom, excitement of driving, etc. I could go on and on. I am so lucky, I had all that and more! The bad - I miss him more and more each day.

The good - I have such a loving family, wonderful husband and sons – the bad --- there isn't any now!!!

Kelly lives in Clearfield, PA with her husband, Steve, and they have been married for 32 years. She has two sons, Justin age 29 and Craig age 25. Craig is getting married in July. She works at their local hospital in the Business Office and her husband is a teacher at the Greater Johnstown Career and Technology Center.

Thoughts of Healing
Nancy Long

Some things I've come to realize since my diagnosis, surgery, treatments, etc:

1) There are so many people going through similar experiences, but I was never aware of it before it affected me...

2) I have started scrutinizing other women's breasts and asking myself, are they real? Are they expanders? Is that a size that I'd like to be?

3) I don't mind not having nipples: I don't worry when I shiver that I have to cover up to maintain my modesty. I'm not sure I even want to have them tattooed on later because I like wearing light colored shirts without worrying that I'm "showing through".

4) You have to do your own research, know your own body, and demand that your care-givers explain everything to you clearly, as many times as you need to hear it.

5) Drains are truly annoying to have to deal with. Ugh.

6) Palmer's Cocoa Butter Lotion is a wonderful, soothing, healing lotion for after radiation (and probably any other time your skin needs to be babied).

7) Having support is vital whether it is friends, family, patients you meet along the way, online forums, chats, support groups, etc. I don't know how I would have gotten through this without my family, especially my mom and my sister.

8) As my bracelet says, "Stay positive" "Attitude is Everything". I live those words, through this journey and, I hope, in all of life.

Nancy lives in Bellefonte, PA. She has three children and as of June 2011, one grandchild also. But don't call her grandma! She's far too young for that moniker. Nancy interviewed with a local government office on her due date with her oldest child, got the job and still works there...um, a few years later.

We Are Here
Dolores Magro

At the PA Breast Cancer Coalition, we advocate for all women and their families across the state. Our legislative victories have created changes that provide mammograms for uninsured women, insurance coverage for reconstructive surgery after a mastectomy, free treatment for breast cancer for uninsured and underinsured women, and funding for researchers in Pennsylvania working to find a cure.

But we are also here to advocate for women who might otherwise fall through the cracks in the health care system, who don't know about available resources or how to access them. Every week, every month, every year we hear from women who need guidance about how to navigate their way through an overwhelming maze of obstacles to medical care. Each time we pick up the phone we know that on the other end of the line there might be a woman whose insurance company doesn't want to cover the procedure that her doctor wants her to have. Or maybe her job is in jeopardy if she has to take time off from work for treatment. Or she has no health insurance and doesn't know there are programs she might qualify for. It is not unusual to hear the caller say "I've asked everyone for help. You are my last hope."

Some days we are providing information about national, state, or local agencies that will provide the service she needs. Often we are explaining a complicated program in a way that makes it seem less intimidating and more accessible. At other times we can be a reassuring voice providing a personal touch in a world of voice mail and computer-generated phone responses.

We were here for Kathryn, whose doctor wanted to perform an MRI on the opposite breast before her mastectomy. Her breasts were too dense for an accurate reading from a mammogram and the MRI would help determine if there was cancer in the other breast. The insurer was not willing to pay for the MRI; however, they would cover the cost of removing the opposite breast if she chose to do that as a precautionary measure. Maybe there was cancer in that breast and maybe there wasn't. Kathryn didn't want to take any chances. Since she couldn't afford to pay for the MRI out-of-pocket, she was prepared to have both breasts removed so that she could sleep at night confident that any and all breast cancer had been removed. Her surgeon's office called the PBCC three days before the scheduled surgery and asked if we could intercede on her behalf. We immediately called, faxed, and emailed the medical director and the CEO of the insurance company. The next morning the company reversed their previous decision and covered the cost of the MRI. Results of the MRI found that her opposite breast was healthy and Kathryn was spared unnecessary additional trauma.

We were here for Ida, who had found refuge in a shelter for abused women. A mammogram at a clinic detected breast cancer and the shelter's medical advocate began a search for treatment. The challenge she faced was that Ida was at that time an undocumented resident and ineligible for many of the programs offered to U.S. citizens. After three weeks of phone calls across the state, the advocate was referred to the PBCC. We didn't know how or where we were going to find someone to take care of Ida, but we were determined to make it happen. After some diligent outreach we learned that she qualified for emergency care only, limited because of her status to what was considered "lifesaving." The PBCC explained that a mastectomy and chemotherapy should indeed be considered lifesaving and Ida was on her way to surgery and recovery.

The Breast and Cervical Cancer Prevention and Treatment program (BCCPT) is the Commonwealth of Pennsylvania's program providing full, complete medical care to uninsured and underinsured women who have been diagnosed with breast or cervical cancer. At the time that Diana was diagnosed with breast cancer, her application to BCCPT was denied because she had sufficient health insurance. However, long before treatment was completed she reached the maximum limit of coverage through her policy. She could barely continue to keep up the premiums, let alone pay for expensive procedures. Despite her earlier experience, we encouraged her to reapply for BCCPT. Her appeal was approved because the new situation changed her status to "underinsured." Diana continues to have full coverage of all her medical needs through BCCPT.

We talked with Florence two weeks after she had stopped taking her daily prescription medication when the cost of the co-pays became overwhelming. When Medicaid denied her appeal for coverage, she reached out to her senator's office and they referred her to the PBCC. We helped Florence to apply for a Patient Assistance Program through the pharmaceutical company that manufactures her medication. We urged her to alert her doctor immediately that she had stopped treatment due to the cost, and to request a one-time supply of the medication to use while she waited for assistance approval. Her doctor's office was able to get 120 capsules for her from the manufacturer. That supply covered her needs until the assistance program paperwork was completed and went into effect for Florence.

We want these women to be able to focus on fighting their disease and getting and staying healthy. If we don't have the information right at our fingertips, we promise to do the searching for her. And then we do it. They don't need to be spending all day searching the internet and making phone calls to find the help they need. We put time and energy into finding resources because we know there is a real person waiting to hear back from us. That realization motivates us to keep looking until we find what she needs. We don't ever want to call a breast cancer patient back and say "I'm sorry but we couldn't help you." Instead we keep up the search until we can say, "I've found the organization or program that will help you." That moment is as satisfying and rewarding as you can imagine. But for every one who reaches out to us we worry about the other women she represents. There may be countless others who don't realize that there is still another place to turn after they hear the word "no." Or they may be just too sick or too defeated to continue to look for another answer. These are the women we continue to fight for with legislation and with funding for breast cancer research. Until one of those researchers finds the cure and we can look back on breast cancer as a thing of the past, the PA Breast Cancer Coalition will be here. We will be here to speak for these women, to fight for them, and to support them along their journey.

Dolores is Director of Patient Advocacy & Conference Development for the PA Breast Cancer Coalition. She lives in Clifton Heights, Delaware County PA and has two grown children, Jennifer and Michael. She is a singer/songwriter and volunteers with Musicians On Call, a program that brings live music to the bedsides of hospital patients. Dolores is also an avid Phillies fan and enjoys going to as many games as possible.

Emerger
Ovie Marshall

My name is Ovie Marshall and I am a breast cancer emerger!
Nothing like I used to be! God Bless!

I am a two time breast cancer survivor. I lost my Mother
when I was four years old to the disease. I've also lost three Aunts
and my sister over the years and in 2005, while nursing my fourth
child, I found a lump in my right breast. I had always been on top
of my health, especially my breast health, because of my family
history with it. But, because I was nursing, I wasn't seeing the
doctor at the time for my breast checks because my milk ducts
hindered the testing. I found this lump all on my own and figured it
was probably nothing, because I had been so careful and aware
over the years. Regardless, I went for a biopsy. I was confident the
doctor would call me days later and tell me I was just fine.

I received the call the day before the fourth of July. I saw it
was the hospital on the caller I.D. before I answered and something
inside me knew the news was not good. I will never forget that
phone call, no woman does. I thought that this was impossible. The
doctor must have made a mistake. My children were so little at the
time, I had to hold my emotion in. I wrote down appointment times
to see the doctor in crayon.

My husband called me on his way home from the golf
course that day. He wanted to see if I needed anything from the
grocery store. I couldn't even talk. I had seen so many people on
my side of the family battle this, I knew what I was up against. I
had the choice of doing chemotherapy, but opted out, since this
was just one lump and had not spread. I had a double mastectomy
and was tested for the Braca 1 Cancer Gene, because my family
history of breast cancer is so strong. Oddly enough, I tested
negative for the gene. This answer was not satisfactory for me
though. I am an advocate of doing it right the first time. I would do
everything in my power to stop this. In 2007, cancer showed up
again in my lymph nodes. I was convinced the Braca 1 Cancer

240

Gene test had given a false negative. I traveled to Sloan Kettering and got a second opinion. It was worth every penny.

The genetics department contacted me and asked if I would be interested in sending a sample of my DNA to France. This testing would be done at my expense, but France had a different, more advanced way of testing for the gene. I of course said yes, and after $350 of my own money, the results came back positive for Braca 1. This changed everything for me. I contacted Myriad Laboratories and they retested me, with the sequencing deletions France had found. Now, Myriad and other labs in the United States test for Braca 1 like France and other European countries do. Now, insurance pays for this test. In just a few years, we have come a long way with Braca 1 testing, but it is important to be persistent sometimes. I was mad it took so long to get the answer, but at least I knew the truth. My whole family was retested and all came out positive for Braca 1. There is a 50/50 chance my daughter can get the gene and I am always thinking about that. I think about the steps I will take when she is older to prevent her from going through this. Prevention is so important to me.

I am cancer free at this point in my life and give all the Glory to God, as he is the ultimate healer. I live to help others by being an advocate of taking charge of your health. When I was diagnosed, I worked part time at my husband's chiropractic office. We found a new passion in our lives to help others prevent cancer. Now, I lecture with my husband to groups and organizations on wellness and detoxification and how products we use can contribute to this disease. Just as my Husband helped me through my cancer, through nutrition and detox, we are helping others. We opened Vitamin Doctor Wellness Center in Greensburg, PA, a place to go and get nutritional advice based on blood work. We talk to our patients about hormones in your body and also important skin care. We are sharing information with others, hoping they take some notes and use it now, or perhaps later, but hoping that they use it when they need it.

I made sure to keep a journal throughout my journey. I encourage others to do the same. It really helped me through the process. I really should have taken pictures. It is an amazing feeling to go back to what you wrote, as you reach three, four, five years out. You read these journal entries and see how strong you feel now. Your hair really does grow back, both literally and figuratively. I can see how scared I was, what my first chemotherapy was like (the second time I had cancer), what the nurses were like, and who visited me. I am so inspired as I go back and read.

Aside from our Vitamin Doctor business, I also have a therapy dog. His name is Duke, a black lab. Duke was around for my bout with cancer and now, I take him around to visit others during their treatment. I take him around to waiting rooms and sometimes nursing homes. I think that is something I never would have thought of doing. Also, my family is very involved in the Westmoreland Breast Cancer Walk. Duke is in attendance at this event, and the dog population seems to grow each year. The dogs join us in the walk, wearing their pink scarves on their collars to show their support.

In my eyes, you can be the victim or the victor. You can live in failure or live in faith. You can be defeated, or you can fight. I chose to fight. I emerged. My family grew closer and stronger. I had close friends that cooked meals for me and prayed for me. Life is good; we are all still here. I believe I am cured by His stripes! No weapon against me shall ever prosper! Fear is just faith in the negative, so we fight for another day! And never give up hope in each other to share words of advice and encouragement and tears of losing loved ones that enable us to persevere and be the light in the darkness for others that walk this road with us.

Ovie Marshall
Assisted by Taryn Noll

Ovie Marshall believes in passion for prevention. She works at the Vitamin Doctor Wellness Center in Greensburg, PA. She is not only a survivor, but a breast cancer emerger, sharing the light of Jesus in healing, hope and health!

My Journey Through Oz
Jill Massey

On another one of my typical, harried days as a working, middle-aged mother, my life would forever change. The day of my annual mammogram, I sped through my day, mindlessly completing required tasks, not giving my upcoming appointment much more thought other than calculating how much time I needed to squeeze it into my day. I was always in a rush, sometimes forgoing my kids' requests for snuggles and goodbye kisses from my husband, just to get a few more minutes lead time on my day. That was until my "journey" with breast cancer began, which I liken to Dorothy's adventures in the Land of Oz.

When skies turn sea green and trees start trembling, you know something ominous is about to happen. Just as Dorothy sensed trouble with the brewing Kansas storm, I suspected something was terribly wrong when the mammography technician kept returning to ask for "a few more pictures." As I pessimistically expected, the pathologist confirmed I would need more tests. I kept telling myself that it would be ok because that is what THEY kept telling me. "80% of calcifications are benign…only 5% are malignancies…it is unlikely this is anything…" Then, just like the tornado that transported Dorothy to a strange land, the phone call that would change my life's course sucked the air from my lungs. The surgeon said something like "bad news" and "malignancy" then "good news" and "100% curable". 100% curable was really all I heard, probably all I wanted to hear. It was the only potential rainbow I could see in this storm.

Off to the internet I went to figure out how to attain the 100% curable state for ductal carcinoma in situ. Boom! My body house just crash-landed as I read that treatment would likely be a MASTECTOMY!!! I was 44 years old with two young children and a mastectomy was not in my plans.

Just as Dorothy emerged from her house to the curious stares of the Munchkins, I met with the poking, prodding, investigative maneuvers of more technicians than one should see in a lifetime. Glenda the good witch, aka my breast surgeon, helicoptered in with the results. Diffuse ductal carcinoma in situ she said. A simple mastectomy was indicated. Follow the yellow brick road. Like Dorothy, I figured the road would get me "home", back to what I considered my normal life.

Then I met the Tin Woman, aka breast surgeon #2, for more tests and the most mechanical breast exam ever performed by a human. After a lecture on the epidemiology of breast cancer and a prediction of my likelihood of dying from something other than breast cancer after her masterful surgical performance, she announced that I would be granted a mastectomy of one breast. When I tried oiling her rust by discussing a preventative bilateral mastectomy because of my concern for future risk and my young children, she chastised me for even considering prophylactic surgery. I left, wishing her luck on her quest to find a heart!

I scheduled surgery with Glenda the good witch, aka breast surgeon #1, still hoping I would soon awaken from this dream. After a flawless surgery, lots of potent drugs and a bumpy ride to my hospital room, I was status post bilateral mastectomy. The last thing I remember was my husband's voice telling me he loved me and would be back in the morning.

My sleepy bliss was rudely interrupted with a fluorescent light flooded wake up call, coupled with a healthy dose of post anesthesia nausea and an invisible elephant on my chest. That's when I met the Scarecrow. The surgery resident announced his arrival to check my wounds. Only eight hours after surgery, I winced as he removed the dressing, never asking permission. He asked if I had eaten anything, not realizing that I didn't get to my room until midnight and it was only 5am. Not waiting for my response, he commanded the nurse to disconnect the intravenous pain medication and prescribed oral pain medications, the same ones my chart said I couldn't tolerate. Just as I started to protest, he had his epiphany, "oh yeah, you were the late case!" I clarified for him that despite my surgical adventures, I was a MOTHER, a DAUGHTER, a SISTER, a WIFE, and a PERSON, not a case! I told him he could probably be a good doctor some day, if he only had a brain!!!

Enter stage left, Glenda the good witch. She humbly apologized for Scarecrow and promised no return visits. She proudly confirmed that she had effectively doused the wicked witch, my cancer, with her surgical bucket of water, looked into the crystal ball and assessed the future to be bright and proclaimed me safely out of the woods! She would release me to the care of the Oz, aka the plastic surgeon, to get me home sweet home and feeling like my normal self again.

I knew I had arrived in Emerald City when I met the gentle, talented, and patient focused plastic surgeon that would put me back together with reconstructive surgery. He was optimistic and encouraging and promised that I would be BETTER than before when this part of the journey was over. I didn't realize at the time that BETTER was more than just the perky "B's" I had requested. I would discover a deep gratitude for the present and a hope for the future that I didn't fully realize I had lost. After several awkward body drawings, lots of photographs, and a couple of perfectly executed surgeries, I got the physical part of me back, BETTER than before, just as he had promised!

Looking back, I realize that reclaiming my physical self was only the rainbow that transported me to so much more!!! I am in awe of the tremendous knowledge, skill and compassion of the health care professionals that cared for and cured me! I am inspired by the women that preceded me with their battles against breast cancer and heroically laid each brick in the road for people like me to follow. Their stories and companionship gave me the courage to face down my own wicked witch, even though my journey seemed so much easier. I appreciate my loving and supportive parents, brother and sisters that offered encouragement and positivity, even when things looked gloomy to me. I am forever grateful to the few friends I confided in about this adventure for their humor, confidentiality, and willingness to listen. Most of all, I value my precious moments with my husband, without whose unwavering support I could not have made it through this, and my children, who to this day, have no idea of the stories I will one day share with them. I now take the time to listen to their stories, laugh at their silly antics, and just enjoy their presence. I won't leave the house without goodbye kisses. I realize that had this all been just a dream, I might never have understood how truly fortunate I am to have my now AND my future. This is my home sweet home and believe me, there is no place like home!

Jill lives in New Jersey with her husband Ken and children Madison and Alexander and dog Steve. She loves running and spending lazy days at the Jersey Shore with her family and friends.

Lessons for Co-Survivors
Diane A. Matthews

Adversity does not TEST you, it REVEALS who you are!
It reveals not only me, but it reveals YOU—you are a Co-Survivor because you help cancer patients survive!

This story does not focus on me, the patient, it focuses on YOU, the Co-Survivor.

Having cancer revealed <u>many</u> things to me, but there are three lessons that I learned that I would like you to remember—these are lessons of vital importance to all co-survivors!

Lesson #1: Cancer PROFOUNDLY affects Co-Survivors.

In my case, I believe it affected you more than it affected me!
I had a mission; you could only stand by, and pray.
You were DEVASTATED by my cancer; I was strong.
You were scared; I was never scared.
You were worried; I never worried.
You cried; I never cried.

My wonderful boys could not say "Cancer" for months. My Mom cried; my sisters cried. My friends worried.

I never doubted that I was a survivor.
We all need to remember…..Cancer PROFOUNDLY affects Co-Survivors.

Lesson #2: If you hear that someone has cancer, don't be afraid to ask them about it!

247

Say, "I heard you were diagnosed with cancer, is there anything I can do?"

If the person wants to talk about it, they will; if they don't, they won't. But NEVER be afraid to ask! I truly appreciate people still asking me today how I am doing!

Lesson **#3:** Co-Survivors are ALL truly amazing!

You helped me TREMENDOUSLY. I was totally unprepared for the outpouring of love, well wishes, gifts, emails, cards, flowers, prayers, and phone calls. I am talking HUNDREDS of emails. I received cards and emails from people I had not seen in 20 years! What strength you provided!

Your support, caring, love and thoughtfulness are the best medicine in the world. Keep up the good work!

Adversity does not TEST you; it REVEALS who you are….

Diane A. Matthews, PhD, CPA/CFF, CFE is the Associate Dean for the School of Management at Carlow University in Pittsburgh, PA. She will celebrate her sixth year of being cancer-free on June 16, 2011. She lives in Allison Park, PA with her husband, Bill, and their twin sons, Brad and Nick. You can reach her at damatthews@carlow.edu.

The Bright Side
Phyllis Maurer

For me, breast cancer had a bright side. No hair? Well, that meant I didn't have to buy shampoo! It also meant I didn't have to shave my legs, and what woman wouldn't enjoy that! Because of my weak arms after treatment, my husband had to help out around the house. Eight years later and he still makes the bed. Now that is what I call wonderful!

Let me start from the beginning. In August of 2003, I felt a lump in my breast. I assumed it was probably a cyst and thought not too much more of it. I knew that if it was something to worry about, the doctor would take care of it when I went for my mammogram scheduled for the following week. Well, it was not just a cyst. I was diagnosed with breast cancer and no more than seven days after my diagnosis, I was starting my treatment. The medical world has a come a really long way in recent years and this really put me at ease.

I was given the option of being a part of an experimental chemotherapy group. My doctor explained that I would only go through four rounds of chemotherapy with this experimental drug. "Only four rounds of chemo? Count me in!" I told him. And so I began my treatment, started the experiment, and was on the road to survival.

I had wonderful people surrounding me with support during my treatment. I believe that everyone you meet in life leaves an impact, positive or negative. I am lucky to have met many people that have been very positive influences in my life. I do not like to be around depressed people because I am such an upbeat person myself! I believe that the optimism and humor I found throughout my surgery came from my mother. My mother was a strong woman. She was not someone who drowned in self-pity. Instead, she held her head high and did what had to be done. It was from her that my whole family learned to keep positive attitudes and let humor heal us.

My treatment was a lot harder on my husband, Ron, than it was on me, and I think is true for most families. It is always harder on the ones who love you. Ron had lost his first wife to breast cancer, and as history appeared to be repeating itself, he began to worry. He stuck by my side every step of the way. He went to every mammogram with me. He sat by my side during my chemotherapy and throughout my radiation. He washed my hair after my surgery, because I couldn't put my arm above my head. Despite the fact that he was more scared than I was, Ron really was my rock and going through breast cancer together strengthened our relationship. As time went on, I think he caught on to a bit of the humor that I brought to the situation. He caught the upbeat spirit of my whole family.

My mother always told us, "No matter how bad you think you have it, if you look around, there is someone else who has it worse than you do." She was so right when she said it. When I was diagnosed, I wasn't upset or scared, because I knew I had already lived a good life. I had watched my kids grow up and had experienced life with my grandchildren. I was satisfied with my life, because I had really "lived" most of it. In my mind, I feel sorry for the young people who are diagnosed. My most important charity is St. Jude's Children's Hospital. I do not like the thought of young people losing their lives before they have even had the opportunity to live them. I want to give to those young people and help them beat their diseases so they can live as good a life as I have had the opportunity to live.

Over the course of my treatment, I trusted God. Any way it turned out, I knew I was going be in a better place. If at the end of it all I was still here on Earth, then that would be great. I could continue my wonderful life with my husband, children, and grandchildren. If it didn't work out, I'd be with God, which is where I always plan to end up.

God sends us messages and guides us to where we are meant to go. To me, breast cancer was just another one of those messages sent from God and He would be guiding me every step of the way. At the time of my diagnosis, I worked in a factory. My co-workers were a great support for me. We were all very close and as I went through treatment, they started a prayer chain for me. It is always good to have God on your side.

I had many positive things come from my breast cancer journey. I was already very close with my family, but our bonds grew even stronger. My husband and I let our relationship grow stronger as well. I also decided to take my life in a new direction with my job. When I was diagnosed, I was working in a factory that produced computer bags. In 2005, the plant closed down, and I suddenly felt the motivation to go back to school. I graduated two years later as a medical assistant and began working at the front desk of a urology office. While I dislike those constantly ringing phones, I really like to talk to the patients. I know how nice it must be for them to see someone who has survived. It is especially nice to be able to pass on what I know lies ahead to others as well. I am not sure what motivated me to go into the medical field after the factory closed, but I am very glad that I sit behind that desk today.

Maybe having breast cancer is the reason that I work in that urology office. Maybe breast cancer is the reason my family bond is so strong. Maybe breast cancer is even the reason why my husband still makes the bed today (because that is pure magic if you ask me). The reason my life is like is it today does not matter to me. Like I said, God works in strange and mysterious ways, but He always has a plan. I am thankful for the life that I have lived and the life that lies ahead of me. Breast cancer was a part of my life, but it was not my whole life.

Phyllis Maurer
As written by Taryn Noll

Phyllis Maurer still works in the medical field. She enjoys time with her husband, children, grandchildren, and great grandchildren. In my life after cancer, the glass is still half full.

Out of the Mouths of Babes!
Sally Mcaneny

My dearest friend Nancy and I were undergoing chemo at the same time. One weekend she and her family, including grandchildren, came to visit. We decided to get dressed up and go out for Sunday brunch. Of course Nancy and I put on our wigs. We were sitting waiting for the others when her 3-year-old grandson remarked, "I guess we're going someplace. Everyone has their hair on."

Sally is a retired science teacher living in Boalsburg, PA.

Authors note: This is short and sweet, and one that makes me laugh time and time again!! Thank you, Sally!

My Journey
Terri McCabe

In January of 1988 I was diagnosed with Breast Cancer. After the initial shock of the diagnosis, I decided that I was going to beat this thing. Single and determined, surrounded by my parents and my surrogate second family: Dorothy, Meg and Susan Helander, I began the first leg of my journey.

On March 18th, 1988 I underwent a lumpectomy. A few days after surgery, my oncologist shared with me that I might not be able to have children as a result of chemotherapy, and this information hit harder than the diagnosis itself. Stage two of treatment meant six months of chemotherapy and six weeks of daily radiation. In the fall of 1988, with the support of family, friends and wonderful doctors, my treatments were complete.

In May of 1995 I married my loving, supportive husband Matthew. In March 1996, our miracle baby Allison was born. Life was GRAND!

One day in the spring of 2008, after substitute teaching a weight lifting class, I met this amazing woman, Lynda Miller. Lynda and I began to chat and she mentioned she was training for the Breast Cancer 3-Day. I told her how many times over the years I considered doing this walk. As we talked, it became clear that this was the year for me to walk. It would be a celebration of being cancer free for 20 years and I was ready to walk as a *Titsy Chick*. We trained, raised funds, trained and raised funds…. The Titsy Chicks were prepared to take on the 3-Day walk in October 2008.

This 3-Day was a life-changing experience. Family, friends, and strangers supported each and every one of us. During these three days, I bonded with these ladies, other walkers, and fellow survivors. The finish line was the highlight of my three-day journey! As we lined up to enter the stadium, the Titsy Chicks (minus one chickie - me) lined up with other walkers, and I lined up with the survivors. As the survivors began to enter the stadium every single walker took off one shoe and held it up in the air to salute us survivors. That was all I needed to see; I no longer held back tears that had been bottled up in me for 20 years.

In January 2009 I was diagnosed with breast cancer again. I was scheduled for surgery on March 18 (yes the exact same day as twenty years ago) until an MRI determined more cancer in that same breast. I underwent surgery on April 14, 2009 and finished my treatments on May 3, 2010. I am now ready to put this all behind me and start training for my second 3-day walk in Philadelphia.

I will walk this October celebrating a year of cancer freedom. To those who have supported me emotionally and physically during my most recent bout: the prayers, calls, cards and visits meant more than words can express.

I'll leave you with a few thoughts...

"So if there is a purpose to the suffering that is cancer, I think it must be this: it's meant to improve us."

"An individual doesn't get cancer - a family does."

"Cancer is not a death sentence, but rather it is a life sentence; it pushes one to live."

"Acknowledge your gifts and be grateful for everything. To look at life with gratitude is to clearly see opportunities. Even at those times of the greatest challenges, with gratitude, any difficulty can be transformed into a blessing, into a meaningful lesson of growth."

"Above all, do not lose your desire to walk. Every day I walk myself into a state of well being and walk away from every illness. I have walked myself into my best thoughts, and I know of no thought so burdensome that you can't walk away from it… If you just keep on walking, everything will be all right."

rriMcCabe

Terri is married to a wonderful husband Matt, and they have one daughter Alli. She loves to spend time with my family and friends, in California, Canada, Avalon and Florida. She is health enthusiast and enjoys reading and time on the beach.

My Story
Eileen McLaughlin

I am a four time cancer survivor. I can say I am a 22 year survivor, a 10 year survivor and a 6 year survivor. I feel blessed to be able to tell you a little about my experience. I hope my story will help just one of you feel better or encourage you to have your tests done on a timely basis.

I had my first breast cancer in 1989. I had surgery followed by 37 radiation treatments. I was lucky I didn't have to have chemo. The doctor told me I was too young and the side effects would be worse than the results. I was okay with this and I went on living and going for my yearly mammograms and pap tests. I was always after my friends and family to go have their mammograms and pap tests. I probably became a nag when I knew someone didn't go for their tests.

After five years, I thought I was in the clear. Five years went into ten years and when 12 years was up in 2001, I got a surprise. I had a bad mammogram. I had breast cancer again. The same breast, but a different kind of cancer. I went through chemo but no radiation. I have to thank my family for the support I was given during this hard time. I also had many prayers which offered more support. I worked every day. I felt that going to work every day was my mental therapy. I did not sit at home and think about what might be or what could be. I had to keep my mind on my job. My customers where so concerned about my health. This gave me the encouragement to continue going to work each day.

The longer the treatment went, the harder it was to get up and go into work. Several times the girls would take one look at me and tell me to go home. Some days were hard but I had the best coworkers anyone could wish for. I also had the support of my family when I came home from work. Not too much got done at home but I knew it would wait for me. One of the girls said to me, "This is one time in your life you can milk everything and not feel guilty." I really thought about it but I tried to pull my own share of the work. I lost my hair so I wore a dark brown wig to

256

work. After my hair came back, I went to work without my wig. I took the wig with me just in case. One of the girls came to work and was so shocked when she saw me; she forgot to lock the door after coming into the office. We all had a good laugh at her shock. Nothing ever shocks her. I did get her for a change. The girls told me not to wear it. I was working in my office that day and several customers wanted to know if I was working. The girls sent them into my office. Some of them did not know me with my silver locks.

I made it through the chemo. I continued to get my yearly mammograms and pap tests. I made it all the way to spring of 2005. I had my pap test. The results came back abnormal. I was sent to Morgantown for a complete hysterectomy. I was blessed; with the surgery I did not need any follow-up treatment. I went home to recover. I was feeling half decent but was still really tired. I went to the doctor in August. Following some tests, I was told I needed colon surgery. I made it through the surgery. It was stage 2 colon Cancer. I had the option to have treatment or not. I opted for treatment. Six months of chemo. Every two weeks at the doctor's office, and then going home with a pump for 44 hours. This would be removed at work and then I would repeat every two weeks for a total of 12 treatments. I kept working with the help of my coworkers and the support of my family. I did not do too much at home after work. But we all survived all for the wear.

I left work one Monday afternoon to attend a meeting in Somerset with my husband, John. John stopped in town to run an errand at a store. I waited in the car. He got out and shut the door. After he shut the door, I heard a beeping. I thought it was something in the car. When John got back in the car, he decided to take the car to the garage. It was only a month old. The salesman didn't know what was wrong so we took it back to the garage. The mechanic and the shop-foreman were checking out the car. I got out of the car and stood close to the front of the car. They looked under the hood and found nothing. So Bill put his ear close to the front tire and slowly turned his head toward me and said, "It is you!" Well, as soon as he said that I knew it was my chemo pump beeping. I proceeded to tell them what it was. Everybody had a good laugh at me. It was worth seeing all the guys laugh. We all need to laugh everyday even though it may be tough. Several weeks later, John stopped in to ask Bill if he had anymore beeping cars. Another good laugh! I finished my six months of treatment in June of 2006.

I never say I am cancer free. I am just clear and hope I will be that way for a long time, even for the rest of my life. I know the support of my family, coworkers and friends along with all the prayers I received is what got me through these tough times. I do believe each time was tough going through treatment, but now that I am finished, I believe I am stronger and see life a little differently, one day at a time. If I can do it, so can you. You see life in a whole different way.

If I can just impress one thing on all of you, go for your tests. Trust your body. If something doesn't feel right, check it out.

Thank you for reading my story. God bless each and every one of you.

Eileen was born and grew up in Frostburg, MD. She is married to John McLaughlin with one son, Corey. She has lived in Meyersdale, PA since she married John. She is a retired Bank Manager with 36 1/2 years of service.

I Am Grateful
Carrie McNulty

I had just returned from life in Northern Ireland, where my husband was completing graduate school. I was finishing my Master's degree in social work and we were living together in an apartment in Pittsburgh, PA. Since I was still in school, I didn't have medical insurance. I noticed a lump in one of my breasts, but I could not do anything about it right away. It started to get bigger and finally, I knew I had to go to the doctor.

The news did not surprise me. Like I said, I had felt the lump before and knew in the back of my mind that it was there. But to me, this didn't make sense. This came out of nowhere. I was young, only 29. I had always been healthy and active. And now, my body was betraying me.

One in eight women get breast cancer and often you don't know when it'll hit you. I think that is the most important thing for people to understand. I quickly learned that I was not as invincible as I thought I was. The worst part was that I had no control over what was happening. I always want to be in control of everything. I had to give up the fact that I would never know why breast cancer chose me. I would never know why this happened. Suddenly, it was like a higher power was telling me, "Hey, guess what? You don't have control over everything."

When I first walked into the oncology office, I was overwhelmed. I saw women covering their heads with scarves and I thought, "I cannot believe this is going to be me."

As my treatment began, I went about it as a business matter. It was all about what had to be accomplished next. I didn't drop out of school. In fact, I kept a 4.0 GPA for the semesters I was in treatment. I also needed to find resources right away (the need to control inside of me), so I Googled local breast cancer support groups. I stumbled upon the *Young Survivor Coalition.* From these women, I gained tons of support, from online discussions to actual conferences I attended. During a conference in Orlando, I was surrounded by over 700 diagnosed women, all under the age of 40.

At the conference in Orlando, we learned to have fun and joke around. At one point, we were in a room full of vendors and walked up to a table of nipples! It is hard to understand if you haven't had reconstructive surgery, but sometimes, you want to try on a nipple and see what it looks like. On this particular day, one of the nipples disappeared. To this day, we joke about who stole the nipple. "Do you have the nipple?" we ask one another. It is nice to joke around with those who know what you are going through.

The women I met through the Young Survivor Coalition are amazing women I will never forget. I wish I could have met them under different circumstances, but I guess this is how we were destined to meet. I believe we will always stay in touch, even when my treatment is officially complete. People do not seem to understand this. To most, it doesn't make sense to keep talking to these women after your active treatment for breast cancer is completed. But for me, it is not that easy. These women helped me and now, it is my turn to help others. I made some really great friends. I do not want to just move on and simply forget about these women. Breast cancer creates this sisterhood between women and I am really thankful to have the close bonds I do with the women I met.

Throughout it all, I had my husband John by my side. We have been together for six years and will be celebrating four years as a married couple in August. He was there to be my caretaker and my support throughout this journey, which has seemed like a complete role reversal. I know it can't be easy, so I try not to drop all the work on him. Together, we made light of a bad situation the best that we could. I believe that you can't take cancer seriously for the rest of your life. You need to have someone you can talk to and joke around with. Otherwise, you will be crying all the time.

John helped me laugh and stay positive. He is bald and has been for a long time. When I lost my hair on day 14 of treatment (when they say day 14, they really do mean you will start to lose hair on day 14), I didn't feel awkward. I could stand next to my husband and feel totally comfortable, the two of us without our hair. We were able to make jokes about my lack of hair. We have a very similar sense of humor. John always made me feel comfortable, even on those days when I didn't feel very pretty. He truly is my best friend and I am so lucky in that sense. We always had a good foundation for our marriage, but now, we are better off and stronger after going through this together.

At first, your life is all about cancer, all the time. But as treatment goes by, you get farther from this thought. Some say that cancer is a gift. I am not sure those are the words I would choose, because I would not give cancer to anyone. Good things can come from breast cancer, though. It just depends on your choices. You can choose to be happy or sad. You can choose to be positive or negative. You can choose to learn from it.

I will say that I learned a lot from the experience. I learned that I was living too much in the past and too much in the future. You need to be appreciative of each day as it passes. If you aren't sure you have a future, you need to be thankful for the moment you are living.

Every day I try to take an inventory of what I am grateful for. I am grateful for my husband who is also my best friend. I am grateful for the women I met and still connect with. And the thing I am most grateful for is the fact that I am surviving. I do not know why breast cancer found me, and I will always be cautious about it possibly finding me again in the future. For now, I am here. I am living in the moment. I am alive. For my life, I am grateful.

Carrie McNulty
As written by Taryn Noll

Carrie is 30 year old a social worker living with her husband and two Boston terriers in Allegheny County, Pennsylvania.

Living With Breast Cancer
Karen Meads

I was diagnosed with breast cancer in July of 2010. It was discovered during a routine mammogram. Shortly after, I learned of several other women who were going through, or had already gone through, similar ordeals. One of my high school classmates had the identical type of cancer and was going through all of the same treatments that I was. I found it incredible that I hadn't connected with these women in many years, and this unfortunate experience that we all went through ended up bringing us back together. Although the news was initially devastating, I was eventually able to gain strength and a positive attitude through the whole experience. I am especially grateful for the support I received from my friends and family.

I feel extremely fortunate to have been treated at Hershey Medical Center. I truly believe that I received the best possible treatment; not only in terms of medical care, but also the support from the doctors and nurses. Because I work in the hospital, some of them knew me as a co-worker before I became their patient. This change in relationship, however, made for bonds that were far more special to me. The breast cancer support group at Hershey has been extremely significant throughout my recovery because I have not had any relatives or close friends diagnosed, so having other women offer their strength and encouragement is very comforting. I am still involved with the support group today, not only for myself, but also in the hopes that I will be able to offer the same consolation to other woman who are in the same situation.
Karen Meads
Assisted by Kelsey Itak

Karen lives in Elizabethtown, PA, She grew up in Hershey, PA and enjoys being outdoors on her front porch swing or walking. She is also involved in spin class to stay active and likes photography. Through here experience with breast cancer, she will be pursuing volunteer work to support other cancer survivors.

The Faith to Heal
Yvonne Mongold

I think the hardest thing I faced after being diagnosed with breast cancer was telling my husband, Bob, who had already lost a wife, his father, and a brother to cancer, and then accept it myself. We cried together for the first several days after receiving the biopsy results.

My husband needed support as much as I did. We were especially grateful to our family, church, and neighborhood dinner club. My husband is retired, but I work full time and had a lot of support from wonderful co-workers. They walked the road with me step by step. June marks my sixth year milestone as a cancer survivor.

Life is not fair and the world doesn't stop because we are facing a crisis. I received chemo treatments on a Friday and the Sunday following was my worst day. My husband stayed up with me all night, encouraging me not to give up. I felt so sick I didn't want to live, but he was a wonderful caregiver and knew what to say and do and also knew what to expect. I had a total of six chemo treatments, one every 21 days and was given three different drugs at each treatment. The first week after each chemo treatment was the worst and I gradually got better until it was time for the next treatment. I lost all my hair a couple of weeks after I began treatments but thanks to the advice of a dear friend, I had purchased a wig ahead of time. I missed work on Friday, Monday, and Tuesday following all my chemo treatments.

Following chemo, I had 37 radiation treatments. The radiation treatments caused me to be weak and tired most of the time. I had radiation Monday through Friday and always scheduled them at the end of my work day so I could go straight home, which was a 50-mile commute.

Being part of a church family is also important and especially when you are faced with a crisis. Being the only keyboardist at my church gave me a purpose to live. I was advised by my doctor not to attend church because people go there more than anywhere else when they are sick. My white blood cell count was dangerously low so I had to exercise extreme caution when I attended.

Although I eagerly welcomed the prayers and desperately needed them, making my cancer public left me vulnerable to those who felt a need to share their story. I stood numb and scared as I listened to their stores. I questioned my faith and struggled with my own emotions.

It is most important to try and keep a sense of humor, if possible. One day on my way to work, I was pumping gas and it was a very windy day. My wig flew off across the parking lot and I had to run after it. On another occasion, I was helping to set up a Christmas tree in our office and my wig got caught in the branches. My co-workers were especially good at making me laugh. I actually looked forward to returning to work for that very reason.

Although my calendar stays full of medical appointments and follow-up tests, I try not to let it control my life. I think the toughest questions I have to answer from people now are "is the cancer gone, did they get it all?" My answer is that I cannot tell you what only God knows, just as you cannot tell me what you may face tomorrow.

God has been with me through this whole ordeal in such an awesome way that it is hard to put into words. I dreaded facing the cancer at first and I certainly did not want to experience another major crisis in my life.

I learned a hymn growing up that expresses it plain and simple: "Many things about tomorrow, I don't seem to understand, but I know who holds tomorrow, and I know who holds my hand".

I could not and cannot make it without my faith and hope in God. It gave me the strength to face each day then and it gives me the strength to face all of my tomorrows.

Yvonne Mongold started to work at Penn State University in 2000 for the Commonwealth College, now known as Office of the Vice President for Commonwealth Campuses and was diagnosed with breast cancer in June 2005. She lives in Mill Hall with her husband, Bob, who is a retired chef. She and her husband have an extended family of seven children, 18 grandchildren, and three great grandchildren, and are actively involved with their church. Yvonne is the oldest daughter of Allen and Arlene McCaslin of Runville. She works full time at Penn State University and enjoys biking and going to waterparks. You can read more about Yvonne and her survival as a cancer patient at: http://heirloomofhope.org.

Not Me!
Judi Moreo

Things like this don't happen to me. Other people, yes. People I know. People I don't know. Not me! Did she really say, "You have breast cancer?" That doesn't run in my family. We have heart attacks and strokes. We don't have breast cancer! But then, she didn't say "we." She said "You." Meaning, "Me."

So it began…mammogram to mammogram to ultra sound to biopsy to ultrasound guided biopsy to surgery – both breasts…on my birthday, no less. At least I woke up to six nurses singing "Happy Birthday."

The follow-up appointment with the surgeon consisted of her explanation of the additional surgery I would need to remove a sentinel lymph node – then a round of radiation treatments.

I thought she said she removed the cancer and all the edges were clean –Was she certain there was cancer in my lymph nodes? Why didn't she remove the sentinel node when she did the breast surgery?

Her explanations didn't add up to anything that convinced me I should be cut open again. I had been led to believe the surgery would consist of a cut an inch long to remove a small tumor. Instead, I woke up to find I had experienced a lumpectomy on one breast, a partial mastectomy on the other. Now, she wanted to cut me open again.

I sought answers. I went to doctor after doctor who told me the standard treatment for breast cancer is the removal of the lymph nodes and then radiation and chemo. Several of my friends were undergoing these treatments – one had neuropathy, one had lymphoma, one died after a long and painful illness.

I am not afraid to die. I've had a wonderful life. What I am afraid of is living an unhealthy life. I decided to do everything in my power to get well. I went for blood tests and a pet scan to determine if there was any more cancer in my body. The first PET scan machine broke down with me in it. I sat in a freezing cold room for an hour and a half while the machine was repaired.

During the second attempt, the lights in the room went very dim so I yelled until the technician came in and told me everyone had gone home except him and me. We finished the scan. I looked at my watch. I had been there 5 hours.

The following Friday, I picked up the PET scan results and returned to my car. Reading the report, I realized the report had my name and birth date but someone else's body. I took the report inside and explained this was not my report. The receptionist insisted it was my report as it had my name and birth date at the top.

I explained to her that I had never had a right breast mastectomy or bilateral breast implants as described in this report. She said she would have a supervisor call me. That call never came.

At my insistence, the oncologist made an appointment with a different imaging company for another PET scan.
I continued my research…seeing more doctors, visiting clinic after clinic and after a month of reading, seeing doctors, watching documentaries on healing and talking with other people who had been through conventional treatments, I made the decision for an "alternative" treatment method.

I prayed for guidance. I prayed for a sign that I was doing the right thing. Then, a friend told me to check out the Natural Healing Clinic in Cedar City, Utah.

The following week, I drove to Cedar City and met Dr. Joe Holcomb. His first words to me were, "Let's see if we can help you heal." After the initial meeting, he put me on an intravenous drip of vitamins, minerals, and trace elements to boost my immune system. I sat for 3 hours with the tube feeding this mixture into my blood stream. Dr. Holcomb administered the drip, left the room, and came back with a book about grief which he suggested I read as my sister had passed away the previous week.

He also noticed I had a stiff neck and was in extreme pain. He said, "On your way out of town, I want you to stop at the chiropractor down the street and get your neck fixed. I made an appointment and he's waiting for you."

The chiropractor, Dr. Neil Logan, was gentle as he adjusted my neck. He also suggested I add Vitamin D3 to my diet.

I asked to use the restroom before I started the 3 hour drive home. While in the restroom, I was continuing to pray about my decisions. Prayer was becoming a 24 hour per day activity. While praying I looked up and saw a beautiful poster that read, "The Power that made the body heals the body. It is the only way." An incredible peace came over me.

Later I was speaking with a missionary friend about the experience. She said when we feel that peace, it is a sign from God.

I knew in my heart I had made the right decision. My choice of treatment may not be right for others, but it was definitely right for me. I made the drive to Cedar City twice a week for six months for treatment. There were extreme life style changes to be made. I changed my eating habits –eliminating sugar, salt, all white foods, all packaged foods, red meat, dairy products, alcohol and caffeinated drinks. I eat mostly raw vegetables and fish and have become very fond of fresh strawberries.

I've taken up exercise. I'd never liked exercise. No one had ever explained to me how important it is to oxygenate our cells. Now I do circuit training, walk, ballroom dance classes and even bought a bicycle.

The most important part of the new life style is boosting the immune system. I have regular vitamin/mineral treatments, colonics, lymph stimulation massages and rest. I regularly reprogram my mind through affirmations, visualization and guided imagery.

Yes, I have to drive 3 hours each way to my appointments and insurance doesn't cover the cost of natural medicines. I have thermal imaging scans every three months to see if there are any changes in my body and I continue with the monthly blood tests with the oncologist. At present, he says I am "cancer free."

I thank my body for the lessons received during this healing journey. I have learned what is really important and what my priorities are. I have also learned to:

* not let people, no matter how expert, rush me into making decisions.
* eat only foods that nourish my body and give me energy
* stop when I'm tired and rest
* spend time with people I love and stay away from those who offer nothing positive to the quality of my life.
* compare the cost of treatment to the cost of poor health
* do things, go places, and be with people because it's what I want

Most of all, I have learned to trust God 100%. I may not understand why cancer happened to me but I know for absolute positive sure that He has guided me through it.

Judi Moreo is a breast cancer survivor, a motivational speaker, and author. Her award winning book, "You Are More Than Enough: Every Woman's Guide to Purpose, Passion, and Power" was written to help women learn to never underestimate themselves. Judi can be contacted through Turning Point International (702) 896-2228 or www.youaremorethanenough.com.

Journey Through Cancer
Shirley Nelms

Throughout my journey, I learned that when faced with an obstacle like breast cancer, you have to fight it with faith more than anything. You must place your faith, not only in God, but also your surgeons, oncologists, and your entire support structure. All of these people serve a purpose, and you must trust that they will successfully help you through. I was especially thankful for my surgeon, Dr. Pamela Scott, my oncologist, Dr. Cheryl Johnson, and the breast cancer coordinator, Cindy Brown. Without these fine individuals, I would not be where I am today. Because of their support, I was able to realize that this is not a battle you can fight all on your own.

During the past year, I found a certain sequence of events just fell into place for me. During my first surgery, they found one bad node. Then, during the second surgery, my surgeon informed me that she had removed 24 nodes and she said, "I held these in my hand, and they felt good. So I'm hoping…" So I told her, "Well you hope, I'll pray." Not long after, one of my drains clogged and the ER doctor told me that I had to see the surgeon the very next day to have it fixed. When I walked into my surgeon's office, Cindy was there. The surgeon told me that I had timed the meeting "just right" and showed me my test results – every node was clear! Cindy hugged me, and of course, we were ecstatic.

There were also several other people who were very special to me throughout everything. I work in a retirement community, which opened my eyes to how many women had already gone through the same experience. There was one woman in particular who would come visit me every once in a while, but was usually very quiet. One day, she came into my office, held my hand, and told me that she had gone through the same thing 15 years ago. After that, she would regularly come down and quietly ask me about my progress; I felt I really formed a bond with her more than anyone. Believe it or not, she is 92 years old. She provided me with a new, optimistic perspective that you can beat cancer and become a survivor. Her support will always mean a great deal to me.

Someone that I had a more humorous experience with was a woman who worked at the prosthesis shop. One night after about a week of having my prostheses, I took it out to find goop all over it. Initially I thought "EW, WHAT IS THIS?!" but soon realized it was the gel from inside. I brought it back the next day, and the woman told me that she had never seen that happen before. She asked if I had a cat; I told her I don't. She asked if I was married; I told her that I'm not anymore. Then she asked if I had a "friend." When I realized what she meant, I told her, "I don't even want to touch this. Do you think I'd be comfortable letting someone else touch it?" We both had a good laugh and she fixed the prostheses for me.

Now that I have successfully completed my surgeries, I am trying to help others through their journeys. Cindy and my surgeon have given me phone numbers for women who are upset or afraid, and I call them to offer support. I have gotten great strength from these women, helping them through everything.

Shirley lives in Downingtown, PA. She is forever grateful to her sons, Dennis and Gregg, for their love and support throughout her journey. It was their encouragement that helped her shape the eternally positive attitude she carries today.

The Power of Pink
Cathy & Taryn Noll

The next two stories are mother and daughter, Cathy and Taryn Noll, and they requested they be together.

Cathy's Story

I never really liked the color pink (too pale and girly for me). Then, suddenly one day, pink is in my life forever.

I was diagnosed in October of 2009 and what a shock! I guess I figured it would never happen to me. After my initial shock, I was rather calm. I needed to get this taken care of and get on with my life. The hardest thing was telling my daughter. She had just started her first year of college and was over three hours away. I wondered who would be there for her when I couldn't be.

Within a couple weeks, I started my treatments. The personnel in the oncologist's office were fabulous. The oncology nurses are great and very caring. On my chemo days, there were always other people getting their treatment too. Everyone was always friendly and upbeat. We always had things to talk and laugh about. It made the time pass faster.

When my daughter came home for her winter break, she took me to my chemo appointments. She got to see all the positive things I had been experiencing. I loved having her home and having someone in the house with me during the day. My husband worked during the day and cooked our dinner every night to help out. Then January came, winter break was over, and my daughter left for spring semester. To help her with her feelings, she started an organization at her college to raise awareness of breast cancer and help other students who are dealing with a loved one or friend who has been diagnosed.

On my last day of chemo, my nurse and I hugged. She wished me well. I told her thanks, and no offense but I hoped I would never see her in that room again. We laughed.

After I finished my chemo, I had a mastectomy and then began radiation. The radiation was the worst part. I went five days a week for six weeks. It made my skin look sunburned. Being tired became my way of life. The hair loss from chemo was a blessing in a way, I didn't have to shave my legs or worry about my hair do.

I am truly blessed to have the family I have. My stepdaughter checked on me and brought her two children over at least once a week to see me. They always brightened my day.

My husband was very helpful during my diagnosis, but now, I have two new men in my life: my oncologist and my radiologist. Both men I have to see every year to make sure I stay healthy.

Through all this I have learned to be patient, something I wasn't known for. You must be optimistic and know you have to fight! A positive attitude is very important. The best thing is the organization my daughter started. It is great for her and the others that can attend. I'm still scared, but I have a lot to live for and know that this is the path my life was suppose to take.

Taryn's Story

I know what it's like to be scared. I know what it's like to cry. I know what it's like to sit in a room full of ordinary people receiving chemotherapy for all types of cancers. I know what it's like when someone is diagnosed with breast cancer. The only thing I don't know is what it is like when you are the one being diagnosed.

My mom was diagnosed with breast cancer in October of 2009. I felt lost. I felt helpless. I felt scared. I was at college, over three hours away, and had no way to physically help her. I couldn't take on extra chores around the house. I couldn't take her to the hospital for treatment. I couldn't even give her a hug. I was worried about her. I was scared of losing her. I suddenly found myself wondering: who would be there for my mom when I couldn't be?

When my mom called me that Monday morning in October, she was not crying or upset. In fact, she didn't seem scared at all. This confused me at the time and it wasn't until I read her own story for this book that I realized what was going through her mind. First off, she was being brave. She knew that this was out of her hands at this point. She wasn't going to wake up tomorrow without cancer. She had no choice but to fight this with everything she had. My mom is a strong woman and I am not sure I truly realized this until her battle with breast cancer.

The second reason my mom was so stoic on the phone that morning had nothing to do with her. It wasn't because she was thinking about the obstacles that lay ahead. She wasn't thinking of losing her hair or losing her breast. In fact, she wasn't thinking about herself at all. My mom acted so brave on the phone that day because she was thinking of me. She did not cry or make a big fuss because of me. My mom wasn't worried about what was happening to her body. Instead, she was worried about me, about how I would handle this. Suddenly, she found herself wondering the same question that had filled my own thoughts: who would be there for her daughter when she couldn't be?

I never understood the bond between mother and daughter. I never had any true desire to understand it either. My mom and I butted heads a lot and our arguments only grew worse the older I got. I saw no possible way for us to ever get along and I assumed we were just not meant to experience the stereotypical mother-daughter best friend relationship. But this experience completely changed us, for the better. The change was not immediate, but over the course of this two year journey, my mom and I found a brand new dynamic in our relationship.

Amidst the medicines, doctor's visits, and chemotherapy, my mom and I both remained strong. I really think we both handled it so well because we were both completely preoccupied. I was busy worrying about my mom. She, on the other hand, was busy worrying about me. We spent so much time worrying about each other, that we ended up forgetting the sadness within ourselves. My mom had been supportive of me countless times in my life before this point and I had been there for her plenty of times as well, but this time was different. For once, we were both invested in the situation. We kept each other on our feet. We were there for each other and it was this constant push of support from both sides that made the difference in our relationship.

As my mom went through treatment, I kept a journal. It was for no one's eyes but my own. I wrote anything and everything that came to my mind. Writing has always been an outlet for me and this experience was no different. I remember writing about taking my mom to one of her chemotherapy treatments over Thanksgiving break. Walking into the oncology office gave me chills, but I tried to hide the fear I felt inside:

> Over my break from school, I took my mom to her chemotherapy treatment on a Monday afternoon. It was so eerie as I walked through the automatic door and stood in front of the elevator I had stood in front of so many times (my pediatrician was right down the hall), begging to go for a ride. Little did I know way back then that the mystery of the floors above us was better left unsolved. Today, we would ride the elevator. Not because I begged, not because my mom wanted to treat me, but because on the fourth floor was room 407, the oncology room: the room where we would battle it, while others battled it. The room where my mom would spend hours each week, fighting it and talking about it, but never actually saying it's name. I am not a huge fan of elevators anymore.

Now, a year and a half later, I realize that the hospital was not a place to be afraid of. All those days at school I spent worrying about her, all those times I wondered, "who would be there for her when I couldn't be?" were not necessary. My mom was in good hands all along. I went with my mom recently to her port removal surgery. When I went to sit with her in recovery, I saw the way the nurses interacted with my mother. They were always in good spirits and always friendly. They paid close attention to her, even though there were plenty of other patients in the room. They remembered little details she had mentioned in passing; like that I was her daughter who went to Penn State. Most importantly, I saw how they made my mom smile. Even though she hadn't eaten all day, her surgery had run a little late, and she was tired and sore, they made her smile. It was these people who had been here for my mom all those times I couldn't be the past two years.

You can try to plan everything out. I am someone who needs this type of control. The hardest lesson I have learned to date is the lesson I learned going on this journey with my mom. You can plan ahead all you want, but sometimes, things aren't going to go as planned. The important thing I learned is that just because life isn't going as planned, doesn't mean it won't work itself out. You will gain control of your life again.

It happened. So what? At that point, we couldn't change that. But we can change how we live our lives from here on out. Things are back to normal, but it is just a different type of normal. Yesterday, my mom called me excited about a new prosthesis coming out that she can wear with a regular bra, not just a specially made bra with a pocket. She was hoping to go to the boutique later in the day to get measured for it. "Wish I could come!" I said, and I meant it.

Cathy and Taryn Noll are not only mother and daughter, but are also best friends. The two live with the rest of their family in Churchville, PA. Taryn is currently a student at Penn State University in State College, PA. In honor of her mother, she is the President and Founder of a breast cancer organization, The Power of Pink at Penn State. To contact Taryn about her organization, please email her at tnollx3@gmail.com.

Taryn is one of the Pink Ribbon Writers for this book.

If Love Was a Cure...
Jackie Ober

In 1997 my husband Leonard was diagnosed with melanoma. Six months later I was diagnosed with breast cancer. We couldn't believe we both had cancer. Len was there for me as I was there for him. When one of us was due for another chemo treatment and our blood count wasn't what the doctors wanted to see, home we would go with a vial of neuprogen, which would give our blood count a boost. If I needed it, Len would give me the shot, and if he needed it, I would administer the shot.

The most important thing I learned from this experience was how to let people care for me. I would do anything to help someone, but found it difficult to accept caring words and help from friends. In the midst of our predicament, I discovered what I had been missing. Len often said, "If love was a cure, we would both be well now." Love and support got us through. Kind smiles, jokes, and laughter all helped, too. I lost Len in 2001, but I remain strong and alive with his love in my heart.

It has been 13 years since I heard the words, "You have breast cancer." I have moved to PA to be near my grandchildren. Joining PBCC has been a way for me to support the cause of curing breast cancer. In 2002 I participated in the breast cancer 60-mile walk. Now I am training for the 2011 Susan G. Koman 3-Day walk. It's another 60 miles, but it's worth the effort to help the cause in any way I can. I support the saying, "Save the TaTas." I promote the importance of early detection with self exam and regular mammograms. Although it was too late for me and I lost both of mine, I feel it was worth it to be alive.

Jackie moved to PA in 2002 to be with her two grandchildren, Tyler and Ashley. She has a wonderful time doing things with them...bike riding, movies and crafts of all sorts. She has two grown daughters, Renee and Kimberly. Kimberly's husband Todd is a dedicated son-in-law who plows her driveway, and is there when help is needed. Jackie acquired a dog in January 2011 named Buster that also keeps her company, and very busy. Jackie works part time as a Dietary Aid.

What Does it Really Mean to Say "I Do"
Dolly O'Leary

You really don't know what you are going to go through
when you say your wedding vows. Who thinks about what the
phrase "through sickness and health" entails" when they are first
reciting during their marriage ceremony? But after a lifetime of
living with fibrosystic disease and enduring a double mastectomy
to fight breast cancer, the phrase took on a richer meaning for me.

When Rich and I married in 1971, I was a widow with
three children. Six years later, we had a child—and 25 years later
we divorced. We remarried in 2000 and I remember him saying
that as soon as we said "I do," I would be covered on his health
insurance (this was very important to him).

I found out that it was just as important to have Rich as my
husband.

Seven years after we remarried, I went in for my six-month
mammogram when a suspicious mass was found. Five days later I
had a biopsy. When the doctor called me two days later and said
that they had found a carcinoma I felt like I couldn't breathe. I had
the wits about me to get the doctor's name and phone number,
called my husband and asked him to call the doctor and get some
details. "Don't worry kid," Rich said; "we'll get through this
together. Remember, it's just you and me, kid." Those words
calmed me down as did some comforting words from a neighbor
and my oldest daughter.

As it turned out the mass was located under my right nipple
and couldn't be found by self examining. The doctors couldn't
even feel it after knowing it was there. From that point on our life
was one doctor appointment after another and lots of tests. I was
very thankful that I had the resources (and health insurance).

I had a lumpectomy, which deleted my nipple, a very small
price to pay. I teased and said that my breast looked like a "ball
headed cue ball." During a lot of the tests that I had done, a
shadow in my lower left lung was discovered. That news threw
me over the edge. I left the surgeons office dazed. I was walking

down the hallway of the hospital somewhere in another world. I found my way to my primary physician, who took one look at me and led me back into her office. She calmed me down enough to get me to stop crying long enough to tell her I didn't want anyone in my family to know and that I just wanted to run away to an island somewhere to try and figure this whole thing out. She called Rich, who wasn't able to get away from work and who asked her to please calm me down enough before letting me drive home. I was 50 miles from where we lived. Before I left her office she again called Rich, so he wouldn't worry, and said I would be OK to drive home.

Five days later I had a pet (positron emission tomography) scan followed up with an appointment with an oncologist. I am very bad about tuning things out! If I don't want to hear something, I just simply don't listen. Lucky for me that Rich was there to hear everything. When you get some news like that, it's so surreal it's like the doctor is talking to you but it must be someone else that is behind you that he is talking about. Rich and I left his office and went home. It had been an extremely long day.

Five days before Christmas I had another biopsy. After it was done I heard one of the nurses say, in effect, that with all the snipping the doctor had done, the cancer had to be gone. I got the results right before Christmas and the nurse was right. What a Christmas present!

My next appointment was with another oncologist. I really liked him as soon as I met him. Good man with a really good bedside manner!

My oncologist gave me the best news ever—I did not have to have chemotherapy. He said that the radiologist would probably try to talk me into radiation, but it really wasn't necessary. We talked and I opted to have a radical mastectomy. Why would I want to keep "My Girls" when they tried to kill me?

My next appointment was with my plastic surgeon. He had done a breast reduction on me a couple of years before. When he walked into my room he looked sad. "Isn't this something," I said to him. "First you're taking it out and now you're going to be putting it back in." We both laughed. It was a long procedure but well worth it.

Before my mastectomy I went to a cancer support group, but I dropped out quickly. I couldn't take the pain of listening to others stories. I wanted so very much to take their pain away, because a lot of cancer patients do not have the support and care that I had.

My husband is my support group, caregiver and best friend. I know he will get me through whatever the case may be. I thank God that my husband is my caretaker. His instinct in every situation that arose is astounding. He always knows what to do whatever the problem is. He never had any training in this area, but you would have thought that caretaking is his profession.

Over the next couple of years I have had several surgeries—including breast reconstruction and a tummy tuck. I do not by any means do well on pain medications. After one of my surgeries I was hallucinating pretty bad. Again, Rich rose to the occasion and made sure that I got the medical attention that I needed.

As I am writing this article I am in the process of healing from another hernia surgery, my fourth in two years, and once again Rich is by my side. I am so blessed to have him as my husband. "Just you and me, kid."

Dolly O'Leary lives in Santa Fe, NM with her husband Rich, her 2 dogs, 2 cats and a tank full of fish. She is retired and has taken acting lessons for several years. She has been an extra in several movies such as Wild Hogs, North Country, and has had some speaking parts in some independent films. She loves gardening, crocheting, cooking & baking. They have 4 children, 9 grandchildren & 1 great-grandson. You can reach her at dollyollieo40@msn.com.

One Hot Momma

When I was diagnosed with breast cancer and was faced with the decision as to whether to have chemotherapy or not, my only concern was losing my hair! My cousin who is a nurse said that would be the least of her concerns, but it was a "huge" deal to me. The only reason the doctor's gave me as to why I should have chemo was because of "my age."

I shared my diagnosis with some of my close friends, family, Pastor KR and Gina, and my co-workers with the agreement that I did not want them to share this with others. Finally, I made the decision to have chemo. Since I was avoiding everything to do with hair loss, I had not even explored what wigs were on the market and it was three days before my first chemo. I remember coming upstairs to an empty family room and the TV was on the Home Shopping Channel – no one in our house ever watches that channel. They were advertising wigs and so I sat down to observe and by the time it was all said and done I decided to order one, didn't tell anyone – I thought, what the heck? The wig was supposed to be delivered in five days, but it came in two, the day before my first chemo treatment. I took the wig out of the box and was amazed as to how much it matched my own hair color and I tried it on – it was perfect! My beautician said I could not have done better if I would have gone to one of those places where they take your hair color and hair style and make you a wig. I knew everything was going to be ok and I could face this chemo with a new attitude. Someone was looking out for me – "Why was HSN on the TV?", "Why did the wig come in two days rather than five?" Thank You God!

Several weeks later as I was sitting at my daughter's basketball game on a Saturday afternoon I was wisping my fingers through my hair, I could feel my hair start to come out. By Sunday afternoon, I knew that I had to try the new wig out – I put it on and went to the store. I felt very comfortable, but everyone kept on staring at me, I wasn't sure why. My daughter said, "It's because you look 'hot'." I thought, "How could a woman who is undergoing chemotherapy and wearing a wig look hot?"

Over the course of the next several months I continued to attend every one of my daughter's sporting events and never missed one. I received so many compliments on my hair (I mean hundreds) and everyone wanted to know who my beautician was... unfortunately, I could not tell them the truth. I could not believe that people did not know it was a wig and by the time they may have figured it out, it didn't matter. Still to this day, I have not shared my breast cancer experience with a lot of people, since that was my way of dealing with it. I am coming up on my 5 year anniversary and I still feel the same way. I attend the "PINK ZONE" day at Penn State Lady Lion Basketball games and other community events, but don't participate as a "Survivor," maybe someday I will change my mind! Everyone has their own way of dealing with things and do what's right for you.

~ Signed, One Hot Momma

Author's Note: One Hot Momma has made the decision to stay anonymous for this publication, but except for the specific details, there are many who can relate to this story, and aren't we all, One Hot Momma?! And to the true One Hot Momma who authored this story, thank you for sharing your story and giving us a smile!

Mom's Story
Jodi Onstead

I am not a survivor of cancer. This story is about my mother. She is an amazing woman with more strength and courage than anyone I know. I have to begin my story by telling of my children. I am the mother of five children a 13 year old, a 5 year old, and 2 year old triplet boys. My boys were born in October of 2008. Mom comes to my home everyday to watch my kids while I work. When Sara started preschool Mom made sure she was there to get Sara to school and also to bring her home. Once I found out I was having triplets I told Mom I will find someone to watch them as they are going to be a handful. She said, "Why, I can handle it, I raised six children of my own". Mom was diagnosed with breast cancer in 2009 at the age of 73. While most people would let this get them down or become depressed my mother did not. She turned to her faith in God and would not allow this disease to beat her. She had to have the lump in her breast removed and also lymph nodes in her armpit. After this she began radiation treatments.

During this entire process she continued to come everyday and still watch my kids, (the boys weren't even one year old yet), even though she was tired from the radiation. She said I can't lie around and do nothing, I am going to beat cancer it won't get the best of me. I just sat back in awe of this woman who has the faith, courage, and wisdom I only hope to have someday. She selflessly worries and cares for everyone else no matter what her day holds. She is now two years cancer free. Mom still has soreness in her arm that the doctor said may always be there. She is continuing her medicine which she has to take everyday for another three years. My Mom along with being the most amazing person I know is also my best friend. She is truly my hero.

Jodi lives in Berlin, PA. She works as a secretary in a local school district. She has been with her boyfriend Darin for almost 7 years now. She has 5 beautiful children, Ashley is 14, Sara is 6, and she has 2 1/2 year old triplet boys, Carson, Ryan, and Brady.

A Sprinkle of Fun from Tammy...

"A chuckle a day may not always keep the doctor away but it sure makes those times in life's waiting room a little more bearable."
                                        -- Anne Wilson Schaef

A New Winning Invention
Cora Lee Phillippi

A kind of dark humor and camaraderie springs up in the hospital after breast surgery...

My roommate and I, after our mastectomies, were trying to think of good things about a mastectomy. We decided that one of the benefits of prosthesis is that if you are really busy and your man is feeling frisky, you can hand him your fake breast and say "Here, amuse yourself with this. I'll be with you shortly."

I don't know about other survivors, but I sometimes take my bra (with prosthesis) off for comfort when I am working around the house. At those times, I don't bother to put the prosthesis in the box.

I have a recommendation for prosthesis makers...

Put a bell or buzzer in them like the ones on phones so that the user can find her boob when she has misplaced it in her bra. The problem seems to happen when one has to get dressed and go out for an appointment in a hurry and can't recall where she took the bra off - upstairs? Downstairs? Help!

Cora Lee Phillippi
As written by Taryn Noll

Cora Lee lives in State College, PA with her husband of over 50 years. She enjoys retirement, traveling, gardening, reading and writing. Her current project is helping Hearts N Hands for Japan to raise funds for tsunami/earthquake survivors.

A Pink Ribbon Story
Alexis Pino

It was March 2004 when my Mom had surgery. I was twenty-seven years old. For a long time my Mom had wanted breast reduction surgery, but not a diagnosis of stage 0 breast cancer (cancer was there, but not developed) that would cause her to decide to have a double mastectomy. Because of stage 0, she fortunately did not have to endure the horrible effects of chemotherapy or radiation.

I was used to always sleeping in. Now every morning at 8:00 I would be up to take care of her at home. The first couple of days after her surgery I would feed and bathe her. I never talked about it much with my friends.

We were told it could come back in 1 ½ years, but I didn't want to believe it. I knew she would be okay. No cells have come back.

My aunt Jo was diagnosed with stage 3 breast cancer eleven months after my mother's diagnosis. I questioned – how did this happen? At 33, I am now nervous – will I get it too?

The first couple of weeks my Mom was in extreme pain. But what I have learned through this time was that my Mom's a very strong woman. I think I would have given up. She can take anything on and fight through it. What I wish I would have known before is more about breast cancer; be more educated about it.

The words of encouragement I would give to other caretakers are to do a lot of praying, be strong and pray to God. You must be positive and be strong for the person you are caring for. This was good bonding time for me and my Mom. I also now look at life differently.

The humor that my Mom and I had found together was that there were no bras anymore. She didn't have to buy them or wear them. We laughed together about it.

My mom is seven years in remission and endures no pain anymore. I thank God for that.

Alexis Pino
As written by Diane Weller
(Family story of Vicki Kovatto, Jo Rivera, Miguel Rivera, Alexis
Pino, and Michael Pino)

*Alexis is a teacher for the Hildebrandt Learning Center at Penn
State University. In her spare time she likes to spend time with her
dog, Verdell, and friends. She loves to take walks especially
during the fall season.*

A Big Curveball
Michael Pino

Everything in my body just stopped! That is the way I would describe the feeling I had when my mother told me she had breast cancer. We were at the dinner table and I felt like I could not breathe and I broke down in tears. There was cancer in my family in other areas, but this was my Mom and I didn't want this to happen to anyone, but especially not my Mom!

Although my mother's cancer was determined to be a category "0", the fact that her diagnosis was determined to be a marker for a pre-cancer, it was still a very serious situation.

Mom had decided to have a breast reduction surgery because she had years of back problems, and I knew this was something to which she had given a lot of thought. I guess a son just doesn't want to know these things about his Mom, but she was always very open as a part of life to let me and my sister know what was going on. She showed us the scars and we had a very open conversation about everything that was happening. She is a very strong woman and she felt this would be better in case we had to deal with something like this in our future.

Mom has always taught me a lot and this experience was no different. Her experience has changed my life. I work harder to remember every detail of every day, the small things that were bothersome are no longer important, and I try not to get upset about those unimportant things in life as I may have before this experience.

My Mom is an incredible woman and I want to remember every moment that we share. She did a great job and I feel she raised a great son, not in a bragging way, but her love never faltered. She was always there to encourage me, no matter what I was trying to do, and she offered everything she had to me and my sister. From clothing, to my beloved Tonka trucks, to all the love and encouragement she has offered throughout the years, I am truly thankful.

Tammy asked me to offer words to other sons (and daughters) who may be dealing with a cancer diagnosis with their mother. I would offer this: be grateful for the life that your mother gave you. I often think about how well my mother prepared me for life, the good and the not as good. You can be a stronger person having a good life, and your mother is always there to love you.

My mother prepared me for life, she taught me about all aspects of life and she gave me these gifts so that I can be a better person and help those around me. My mother is the best! There were other kids in our neighborhood growing up that some people would say were "bad kids", but Mom wanted more for us. She did everything in her power to make sure we made the best decisions. And, it wasn't just the big stuff that counted to my Mom. I fondly remember her teaching me how to brush my teeth; it wasn't just 30 seconds, no, Mom made sure we understood why it is important to do the right thing the right way the first time. If I didn't do it right, Mom sent me back again until I made sure it was done right. This is a lesson I learned to take with me from childhood into adulthood and it has served me well.

When Mom was diagnosed, I had to take a good look at myself and believe that God allows these things to happen to help prepare us for life.

I do worry that Mom's cancer will come back; I think that is only natural. Right now my mother is here for me and I will be here for her. I try to enjoy every "nook and granny" of life that we share. Sometimes I record our adventures, like a recent trip to Hershey Park. We never know what might happen and when, and this experience has certainly taught me to be involved with every moment we have with our loved ones.

This whole experience threw me a "big curveball", that is the only way I can describe it. Totally unexpected but full of lessons I will take with me always. Our conversations are a lot more meaningful now, I do not take her for granted, and I realize that life can change in the blink of an eye. Before this, I had a difficult time saying, "I love you, Mom", but I don't any longer. I believe it was God waking me up and maybe asking, "Do you appreciate what I gave you?" Now, I can truly say that I do. God has given me a second chance to get this right, and I am thankful. And, my final thought, I love you, Mom!

Michael Pino
As written by Tammy Miller

(Family story of Vicki Kovatto, Jo Rivera, Miguel Rivera, Alexis Pino, and Michael Pino)

Michael is 30 years old and lives in the Philadelphia area. He has olive skin with black hair and has always had a love for fast cars and auto mechanics. He has his Mother's laugh and sense of humor. He is a fork-lift operator and loves anything that has to do with history.

God Sends Angels
Sister Marie Poland

"Can it wait until I return from Omaha?" The telephone call from my doctor was not what I wanted to hear. I was in the middle of getting my Certification in Spiritual Direction from Creighton University in Omaha, Nebraska. My summer session would start in just about three weeks and this was no time for me to have health problems. The Doctor insisted I see a surgeon immediately. My annual mammogram had shown a lump in my right breast and I needed a biopsy now. When I told her I did not have a surgeon in mind (does anyone?), she gave me the name of a group in Lancaster. I called immediately and saw the surgeon the next day. By the time I arrived at the surgeon's office I was terrified. Cancer can do that to a person and I was no exception. That visit turned out to be the most horrific event of my entire Cancer experience. The doctor, when he saw my tears, asked me what was wrong with me "women do this all the time, it is really no big deal." Well, THIS woman did not do this all the time and this woman was scared out of her mind. As it turned out I left his office with an appointment for the following week but I knew I would never return to that office again. I was in search of a different place to have my cancer treated.

When I arrived home I started thinking a little more clearly and realized that Hershey Medical Center was only a half an hour away. Why hadn't I thought of that before? I went on line and found the number for the Breast Center. When I called, the kindest, most understanding person answered the phone. She calmed me down, she reassured me that I would not have another experience like the one I had just had and she got me an appointment for the very next day. Katherine Love—such an appropriate name—was that angel. Katherine had experienced Breast Cancer herself and she knew how scared I really was. When I arrived for my appointment with Dr. Smith, I once again, became a terrified, crying woman who needed understanding and compassion. I received all that and more from Dr. Smith and the nurses at the Breast Center. The nurse who held my hand while I had my first biopsy was the rock I needed to hold onto at that moment—another angel sent from God. Dr. Smith reassured me and talked to me throughout the procedure. Although I really was unable to relax, I was grateful for their concern. The biopsy results came back the following week and it was malignant. I opted for a partial mastectomy and radiation treatments. I wanted it over as soon as possible. Omaha was now not an option in my mind. I would wait until next summer, I will continue my studies then. I underwent the surgery and a few weeks later began the radiation treatments.

The people at the Radiation Center were also the kindest, most compassionate people I had ever met. After my first visit to the Radiation Center, I went to my car and cried and cried. I did not belong here, it was for sick people, very sick people, I had seen them in the waiting room—would that be me in just a few weeks. Terror seized me. I went home and cried some more.

I finally began to look through some of the literature given to me at my appointment. I didn't even want to touch the bag they gave me—I didn't want this to be real. I knew if I started reading about it, I would have to admit I had cancer and I really did not want to do that. After finally looking through some of the brochures, I found the number of a group called "Y-Me". They said they had a 24 hour hotline for anyone to call at any time they felt the need. Well, it was about 11 p.m. on a Saturday evening and I was feeling pretty alone and very upset and scared. I called the hotline number. The woman who answered the phone was another angel—when I told her I wasn't sure why I called, I began to cry. She soothingly talked to me for over an hour as I apologized for not really knowing why I was crying or why I called. I slept better that night because of her.

When my radiation treatments began, I went back to my terrified mode. I found it hard to believe that no harm would come to me while I lay on a treatment table, naked from the waist up with my arms above my head and a giant machine over my body shooting radiation into me. The nurses and technicians understood my fear and did their best to comfort me—I came to like them all and did get a bit used to the treatments but was very happy when they were done.

My cancer returned two years later in the opposite breast. I can't say I was any less terrified, but I can say I knew I would be cared for. I went through the surgery and radiation again—this time like a seasoned pro. I still had my bouts of tears and fear, but I knew as I walked this journey I would not be alone.

I finally finished my summer classes and received my Certification in Spiritual Direction and my Masters in Spirituality. My experience became the topic for my Integration Paper needed to graduate from Creighton University.

I continue to have my six month check ups and another "spot" was found. Another biopsy done but this time it was benign. Looking back upon my experience I know God had sent Angels to surround me and console me as I journeyed on this path. I came to recognize them in those who cared for me and about me. Now I hope to be an angel for someone else who is in need of that love and concern.

Story Two
NO CHEMO!

Oh, you are so lucky—you are not having Chemotherapy. I heard that phrase so many times during my bouts with Breast Cancer. It is as though not having Chemo meant that my breast cancer was the "easy" kind. I would not be losing my hair, I would not have the spells of vomiting that those with Chemo have to go through. I chose not to have Chemo, after a good deal of research and studies. My reasoning was because at my age the survivor rate was not much higher with Chemo. So, when I weighed all the factors, I opted to go for the surgery and radiation. Of course, I did not know anything about either one.

I soon found out, though. Radiation was not going to be the cake walk I had hoped for. When I first arrived at the Radiation center I was met with a room full of cancer patients, all

294

in various stages of their treatments. Some seemed very happy, engaging in conversations and laughing with each other. Others seemed to be very worried, scared or angry. I took my place among the group, waiting to be called. I didn't want to talk to anyone, I was too frightened. My sister, Kathy, had come with me and was trying without any luck, to lift my spirits. When I finally was called, Kathy was told she had to wait in the waiting room and I would go back with the technician. I had come alone for the pre-visits: the measuring, the CT scans, the x-rays, the markings and the tattoos. After my first visit I returned to my car and began to cry—fear had overtaken me and I couldn't keep up that strong front anymore. I suppose Kathy had sensed that in my voice when she called and asked how it had gone. I couldn't hide my fear—not from my sister, anyway.

She waited in the outer waiting room, while I went into the testing area. There I found another waiting room, this one filled only with patients. We had been taken to dressing rooms and in various stages of undress we all sat with our white robes on waiting to be treated.

My turn came and I was told to lie on the table, remove my arms from the robe and place my arms above my head. There is a certain vulnerability that comes with lying naked on a hard x-ray table with your arms stretched above your head. This would be the position I would have to take every day for the next 35 days of treatment. I wish I could say it got easier as time went on, but it really didn't. I guess I could say I got used to it, though. The technicians working in the Radiation Center did everything they could to make things easier on the patients. They were kind, gentle, understanding and extremely compassionate. I tried my best to keep my own spirits up—I treated myself to my favorite magazine, out to lunch with a friend, ice cream, anything to make me look forward to the next day. I began bringing candy to the technicians every Friday as a celebration of another week gone by—it became a bit easier as I became more relaxed. I did have some "sunburn" effect to my affected breast. This got warmer after each treatment, but never unbearable. It was amazing how patients bonded in the "patient" waiting room. Each patient would encourage another that the next few sessions would be tolerable. We clung to the experience of the others, not knowing what to expect and wanting to hear that things would be okay. After the 35 days of Radiation—on your last day of treatment—you have the opportunity to ring a large bell and declare your "freedom". Each person rang the bell with all the strength they could muster—this was a big step for each one of us.

For many of us, this would not be the last time we rang the bell. I went through the process again two years later on my other breast. This time I knew what to expect and was able to get through without a great deal of struggle on my part.

The lesson I learned from all of this? Never judge how a cancer patient is doing by how they act. The fear and anxiety that dwells inside can be more than anyone can imagine who has never experienced it. Never think that any form of cancer or cancer treatment is minor—it is never minor to the one afflicted with it. Remember to try to lift the spirits of those who are going through treatments or doctor visits. Even a "routine" checkup is never routine for someone who has suffered a cancer experience. And, most of all, be grateful for those individuals who dedicate their lives to helping cancer patients.

Sister Marie Poland is a Roman Catholic Sister in the Community of the Adorers of the Blood of Christ. She is a school nurse in Fink Elementary School in Middletown Area School District in Middletown, PA. She is a Spiritual Director and guides retreats. Sister Marie loves to travel and read.

Pink Rose Inspiration
Nick Pyykkonen

Nick Pyykkonen – Son of two-time Breast Cancer survivor and Nephew of 2 deceased Aunts taken by Breast Cancer

Aunt Carol lost her battle in 1997 and eight years later, in 2005, Aunt Kathy lost her battle as well. Almost one year to the date of the death of Aunt Kathy, my mom, Beth, was diagnosed with breast cancer for the first time. She would fight and win her battle against breast cancer and become a survivor, after visiting MD Anderson in Houston Texas multiple times.

In the spring of 2009 she would be newly diagnosed with breast cancer for the second time. After trips to Anderson once again and the Rose Cancer Center at Royal Oak Beaumont, battling bravely through both journeys, we are happy to say she is now a two-time survivor. She finished her last round of chemotherapy in November of 2009.

My mom continues to battle the after effects of fighting this battle, such as depression. Wanting to take action against this destructive disease, I launched the Pink Rose Inspirational Foundation in October 2007 and incorporated in July 2008 vowing to make the journey through breast cancer easier for patients. This foundation was formed to celebrate life: the life of past victims, the life of survivors and the vision of a normal life as a breast cancer survivor! It was formed to ensure that no husband, son or nephew has to experience the loss of life, and normalcy of life which breast cancer takes from those it affects. After watching my mother go through this disease for a second time and battle depression as she has, it fuels my fire even more to fight back. I honestly do not wish this upon any other person in this world. The emotional toll that breast cancer has on the patient and the family is terrible!

I am glad there are other people out there such as all of you reading this, who want to do something to fight back. I hope that we can make medical and other treatment/support advances to tip the odds of this fight in our favor!

297

Sincerely,
Nicholas Pyykkonen
President and Founder
Pink Rose Inspiration

You can reach Nick at www.PinkRoseInspiration.org

Fore! Life
Geri Reeve

I have had cancer over half of my life. I found my first lump at the age of 28 which resulted in my first mastectomy. I remember the night before I was operated on my daughter climbed up on the hospital bed with me and said "Mom, are you going to die?" That has been my driving force to survive and help other women with children to know you can survive. Unfortunately, I had a second mastectomy 13 years later and that resulted in six months of chemo and five years of Tamoxifin. By the time I had my second bout with cancer, I had become a pretty avid golfer and someone who loved life. Even on chemo, I would go to the golf course and my friends would pick me up in a golf cart to let me play a few holes. Four of those friends, Nancy Lippincott, Mary Ellen Hurley, Suzanne Cummings and Anne Marie Lee decided to get a golf tournament together and donate the money to the American Cancer Society. That was the beginning of the Geri Reeve Open Golf Tournament.

In 1993, we donated $393 to the American Cancer Society. Over the last 17 years we have raised approx $260,000 for the American Cancer Society and the Centre County Breast Cancer Coalition. The growth and continued success of the tournament has been accomplished through the entry fees paid by the golfers, local donations, and a very hard working tournament committee.

The money we raise is truly secondary to my main purpose which is to promote awareness of breast cancer and the importance of early detection. In 2000, we added Centre County Breast Cancer Coalition so that people living in Centre County could benefit and receive some financial assistance for mammogram testing. Without a doubt, someone out there is alive today because of the Geri Reeve Open.

My support does not stop at the golf tournament. Over the years I have been involved with Living Beyond Breast Cancer which is based in Philadelphia, Susan B. Komen's Race for the Cure in Pittsburgh, Susan B. Komen's Drive for the Cure, Relay for Life, Sew for the Cure, Creative Arts through Penn State, and Reach for Recovery. I'm also a past board member of the American Cancer Society and president of the Centre County Breast Cancer Coalition.

We depend on self-examinations, mammograms, MRIs and doctors' examinations to detect breast cancer. Statistically, one out of six women died from breast cancer when I had my first bout with breast cancer. Now that number is one out of nine.

When I heard, "I'm sorry you have cancer". I didn't believe it the first time but when they told me the second time, you are now entering a whole new world. My cancer journey hasn't always been fun and it certainly hasn't been easy. I do believe that modern medicine truly is a miracle. Recovery does not happen in a day, a week or year. I would not be here today if it wasn't for the treatment and support from my family, friends and doctors and especially my little granddaughter...Paige. She brings so much happiness. When I was told the first time I had cancer all I wanted to do was to see my daughter Karen grow up and be happy. Now my vision has changed. I want a cure so breast cancer will never be part of anyone's life. If you have cancer never give up and do the best you can to make the most of everyday.

Geri was born in Washington, VA. She has two brothers, her mother is still living and her father deceased. She moved to Hanover, PA in the early 70's and later to Centre County. She has a daughter, Karen, son in law Chris, and her beautiful granddaughter, Paige. She has had cancer three times in my life beginning at the age of 28 and has spent most of her life involved with helping other cancer patients. She has been involved with Relay for Life since the beginning, Reach to Recovery, Living beyond Breast Cancer, past member of the board for American Cancer Society and current president of the Centre County Breast Cancer Coalition. She feels very fortunate to have a Golf Tournament in her name and the proceeds go to underprivileged and underinsured women in Centre County with donations amounting to almost $300,000.

She admits that the best part of my life now is her little grand daughter Paige. She has brought so much joy and fun to their lives. She gets to watch her grow and learn in swim class, dance class, soccer and the bowling league. She is going to school and reading to Geri as Geri once did to her! Retirement from Penn State as a Financial Aid Coordinator is just a couple of years away and she hopes to spend more time with Paige.

Finding Treasures in Unexpected Times & Places
Margo Reinke

I stared rather incredulously at the little plastic card in the palm of my hand. "Ottawa Regional Cancer Centre," it read. And it had my name on it. I had an oncologist -- and before I knew it, I had two oncologists. But they treat people who have cancer. These little truths that were forcing their way into my brain were all leading me to the one big truth that I had to wrap my head around: I had cancer. Breast cancer. Yes, this was my life these things were happening to. Somehow that little plastic card made it official. Well, OK then. Is it possible to be unsurprised and yet shocked at the same time? After all, my extended family has seen a lot of cancer, including breast cancer. So, not a big surprise. But this was _me_. That gave me a jolt that I felt right down to my innermost fibers.

Back to the beginning. Whatever this thing was that I'd discovered in my breast, there was no mistaking it was most definitely a lump of some sort. The flurry of mammogram and ultrasound, swiftly followed by a biopsy, was followed by what felt like an interminably long wait for the biopsy results. While I went through the motions of everyday life, the question mark of biopsy results never left my mind. I had a bad gut feeling, and the moment I got a call to go see my doctor, I knew what the results were. After all, they'll give you good news over the phone.

Next step: see a surgeon. The surgeon came out to the waiting room, and, looking at a file, called my name. Three women stood up in unison. A friend had gone to the appointment with me to help take notes. A second person seemed a good idea, as doctors' words these days tended to swirl around in my head a lot without really landing anywhere. We had stepped into the waiting room to find another friend sitting there waiting for us to arrive. Thus, three women rising to see my surgeon. Aren't friends wonderful?

Strange as it might seem, one of my questions for the

surgeon concerned a dog. Some time before my life had taken this turn, I had picked out a puppy, which would soon be ready to leave its mother. The dog had been in my plans; breast cancer had not. Upon questioning, the doctor assured me that I'd be able to handle a puppy. I think perhaps he's never raised a puppy. But I proceeded with my plans and picked up my new pup on the arranged date, which happened to be two days before breast surgery. I've been forever grateful that my two sisters in Kingston came to Ottawa to be with me, so I had help. And pet therapy.

My surgeon had told me that I'd need "at least" surgery (a lumpectomy) and radiation. My brain interpreted this in a manner that simply omitted the "at least" part. So when my radiation oncologist told me I'd have to see a medical oncologist (who looks after chemotherapy), I was puzzled. Why did I have to talk to someone about chemotherapy? (And aren't all oncologists "medical"?) But I had myself convinced this was just a step I had to go through – that the medical oncologist simply had to confirm that I didn't need chemo, so I could get on with the business of radiation. Post-surgical pathology reports put an end to that notion and started my education in a whole new language. The language of cancer, with all of its terminology, the ins and outs of treatments and home nursing visits – so many things of the sort you never before imagined learning, especially in application to your own life.

As the time for each chemo treatment would approach, my oldest sister, who was then retired, would come from Kingston and stay with me for about a week. Neither of us has ever been very handy in the kitchen, but her husband, being quite talented in that area, sent pre-prepared meals along with her every time. Hair loss happened fairly quickly, and I began buying hats like crazy. I didn't buy a wig; I was content with hats and scarves. And I learned that there are definite advantages to the low maintenance requirements of baldness – and there's never a bad hair day!

I attended a series of meetings called "Healthy Living for Women with Breast Cancer." Here I met a small group of remarkable women who were also undergoing breast cancer treatment. When these sessions ended, we decided we wanted to continue to meet. Several years later, we're still getting together, having dubbed ourselves the "Treasure Chests." While my friends and family have always been a wonderful support, it's very special to have this group of Treasures, knowing we understand each other, helping each other through rough spots, providing encouragement and celebrating the good things. I cherish their friendship, recognizing that had I not had breast cancer, I would never have met these women.

After chemo came 30 radiation treatments. Daily trips to the Cancer Centre became the routine, with weekends off. By the time all of this was finished, it had been one year and three days since I'd found that fateful lump, and I felt like my breasts had been examined by every medical professional in town. It went along with the raw, vulnerable feelings of the entire cancer experience.

A year after my treatment ended I encountered another wonderful group of women. At a meeting of Breast Cancer Action (BCA), I learned about "Busting Out," an Ottawa dragon boat team of breast cancer survivors who operate under the umbrella of the BCA organization. I was immediately excited about the idea of joining "Busting Out," and since then it has played an important part in my life. Here I found another group offering support, understanding, laughter, fun, fitness, and fellowship. We are, as we say, all in the same boat. And out on the water, in this boat, all is good for body and soul. Being part of "Busting Out" has also provided other new opportunities in my life. In September 2007, 34 "Busting Out" paddlers, along with supporters, travelled to Australia for "Abreast in Australia 2007," an international dragon boat regatta for breast cancer survivor teams. It was an incredible experience, spending three exhilarating, intoxicating days with 1700 breast cancer survivors from Australia, New Zealand, Italy, Hong Kong, Singapore, the U.S.A., and Canada. In 2010 we competed in another international festival, hosted in Peterborough, Ontario. While it didn't include the excitement of travelling to Australia, Peterborough did us proud. They did an outstanding job, welcoming 2000 breast cancer survivor paddlers – with teams from Britain and South Africa added to the mix. Again, the atmosphere was electric. And as in Australia, we paddled our hearts out, we partied, we cheered, we hooted and hollered, we sang, we laughed, we danced. We celebrated life. In a big way. And this, really, is what breast cancer has given me – it taught me how to celebrate life.

Margo Reinke lives in Ottawa, Ontario. She discovered that cancer can have surprising and unexpected effects on one's life, perceptions, and priorities. While many people view cancer survival as an accomplishment, Margo feels that surviving the cancer treatment was the real accomplishment! (However, it is the treatment to which she attributes her current cancer-free status).

Never Giving Up
Tara Ripka

My name is Tara Ripka and I am a cancer survivor. I'm celebrating my 10 year survivorship this year!!!! I'd like to share my cancer story with you.

Ten years ago in May, I felt a sharp pain in my left breast. That's when I first noticed a lump. I was only 27, so I wasn't really worried. A month later, it was my scheduled annual check up. I told the doctor about the lump. They too felt it, but were not very concerned because of my age. Luckily, they did send me for a fine needle biopsy. The fine needle biopsy was inconclusive, so they scheduled me for the lump to be removed. The surgeon too, was not concerned. He said I was too young to have breast cancer. So far, I was not very worried because all the professionals were not worried.

In June of 2000, I had a lumpectomy. Right before I went under anesthesia, the doctor said, "I'll owe you dinner if I'm wrong, it's not cancer, you're too young." Well, that doctor still owes me dinner.

When I woke up from anesthesia, my husband and mother were right by my side. They knew the bad news before I did. I still remember my husband saying, "We're not done yet, it was cancer." That's when it all hit. The tears, the fears. The reality of the fact that I was only 27 and had breast cancer. So now what?

I went home that day to my dismantled home. We were in the process of selling our house and building a new one. My bad news came 2 days before we needed to be out of our home. I had a lot of loving friends and family call and stop by to see me. Seeing my dad for the first time was one of the toughest parts. Seeing him cry and the fear in his eyes was something I'll never forget.

The only good thing about all of this happening when I was in the middle of a move, was the fact that we were moving in with my parents while our new house was being built. There's nothing like being at home when you are sick and having your parents take care of you. When my husband was busy working on the new house, there was always someone there for me.

2

The next surgery was in July. It was a lumpectomy to clear all margins and a sentinel node biopsy. They inject a dye into the breast to see where it travels. Those are the lymph nodes they then take out. At that time, I remember the staff saying I was the youngest person to have this done. I think I still hold that record at Mt. Nittany. But, it is not the record I would have chosen to hold.

I spent the night in the hospital after that surgery. The hardest part of that recovery was the drain tube hanging from my body. I don't remember exactly how long it stayed in, but it was too long. I also remember calling my sister from the hospital when they discharged me and told me to get dressed. I couldn't move my arm and I couldn't dress myself. I was too stubborn to ask the nurse for help, so I called my sister crying to come help me. And of course, she came.

I needed to recover from this surgery before any treatments started. I remember my first appt. with the oncologist. He told me that I'd need chemo and radiation. His first comment was, you will lose your hair. At that time, my hair was the longest it had EVER been. I think the tears started up again at that time.

The cancer was an aggressive cancer, but luckily it was enclosed in a cyst and it did not spread. That was the best news ever at that point of my life!

My first chemotherapy treatment was Aug. 9, 2000. It was my parents wedding anniversary. So I'll never forget that date. It actually went well. I scheduled the treatments when the soaps were on so I'd have something to watch to pass the time.

I did not get sick from the 1st treatment. I was just very tired. A few days later, I remember drinking a soda and I thought it was flat. So I opened another one. It too tasted flat. Then all food started to taste different and not so good. Even chocolate didn't taste right. Now, that made me mad!

I started to feel normal again before my 2nd treatment and went back to working. Then, it was Grange Fair Saturday, I'll never forget that date either.

After my shower, my hair just knotted up in one big hairball. I could not comb it. For every time I tried, it just came out. That was a very emotional time for me. My aunt, who was a hairdresser, lived on the next street. My mother and I went over for a haircut. I wasn't ready for it to be shaved bald, so she just cut it very, very short. I remember crying a lot that day. I probably should have shaved it from the beginning. I had to use a pet lint brush on my pillow every morning until it all eventually fell out anyway.

That's when you and everyone else knows you have cancer. When you are bald, and pale. I hated looking in the mirror! It is just not a good look for women. I would wear a wig when I went out in public. It was a decent look, but boy was it ever itchy! I would wear hats or scarves around my daycare kids and family. The daycare kids were so wonderful through my sickness. I'd have a wig on one day and the next just a hat and they would just say, "Oh, your hair grew back".

My next 2 chemo. treatments didn't go quite as well. I did get sick those times. I slept a lot for a few days after. But, that's what my body needed to get better. By my 4th and final chemo. treatment, my new home was done and it was time to move in. I did not get sick this time. I think I was too busy unpacking boxes this time. I sure did have a lot of help with the move. I couldn't have done it all without my family.

It was probably a month later before I started radiation treatments. We needed to wait for my blood counts to go back to normal. Radiation was a breeze compared to chemotherapy. This was 5 days a week for almost 8 weeks. As long as they were running on schedule, it was a quick trip in and out of the hospital.

The only side effect of the radiation was sensitive skin, like a sunburn.

After all those treatments, I was cured. I have been in remission for 10 years. I now do everything in my power to keep it that way. I have a mammogram every year. I also have a breast MRI every year. I had genetic testing done to see if that was the reason that I had breast cancer at such a young age.

I tested positive for the BRCA1 gene mutation. With this mutation, I am still at a greater risk for another breast cancer and ovarian cancer. With every year that goes by, I have a 5% increase risk of another cancer. With those odds, I had my ovaries removed 2 years ago. That dramatically decreased my risk of ovarian cancer by almost 100% and it also decreases my risk of another breast cancer by 50%. The hardest part of that surgery was instantly going through menopause at age 35. I'm still thinking about having a double mastectomy sometime in the future. I eat healthier than I use to. I exercise when I can. I read every cancer fighting article that I come across. I raise money with my Relay for Life team to help find a cure.

I was lucky enough to be blessed with 2 beautiful and healthy girls after my cancer. I will do everything in my power to keep myself healthy and I will continue the fight for a cure for their future.

If you know someone going through cancer, your support truly means so much. A hug, a phone call, a card, helping with childcare or household chores. Cooking for the family or helping with transportation are all things you can do for support. No one should have to go through cancer alone. The community support through the Relay for Life means so much to me as a survivor. I thank everyone here for that support. Let's never give up the fight!!

Tara lives in Bellefonte, PA with her husband Todd and two daughters, Shaylin and Sadie. She is a stay at home mom and a part time substitute teacher. Tara can be reached at tararipka@yahoo.com

A Pink Ribbon Story
Jo Rivera

My routine mammogram had been delayed. When I look back now as both a victim of breast cancer and a survivor, I cannot help but question – what would have happened if the mammogram had been done earlier? I am trying to let go of questioning this, but it is hard.

I was given the news that I had an aggressive, fast-growing cancer. I was in shock. No one else in my family had ever been diagnosed with breast cancer of the same type and stage as mine.

The time between August 2006 and February 2007 was eight months of not being able to work, but undergoing thirty-five radiation treatments and eight horrible chemotherapy treatments. During chemo I hoped to God I never had to go through it again. It's awful – I would not wish it on anyone. Although a nurse myself, I knew from my experience that I could not administer chemo to patients.

I came to know what days I would not be able to get out of bed and what days I could go shopping or do other things. It was down to a science – I just knew my body that well. I also frequently felt the need to coat my stomach. Not in an appetite satisfying way, but in a way that made my stomach feel right. I craved milkshakes and hamburgers – not a normal thing for me.

I learned to take life one day at a time. Each day I looked forward to crossing off another day as I went through my journey of treatments. Each day crossed off made me hopeful that I could do one more. During this time I also learned to say "no."

I have been in remission for five years and back to work at the hospital. I talk with patients about chemo and radiation. I tell them it is not all gloom and doom. There is hope and there is treatment. My best medicine, however, was my breast cancer support group. Being part of this group was the best thing I've ever done during this time of my life. It was the only time I could laugh. We'd laugh about our wigs, our bald heads and lots of other little stupid things. My joke became "I have hair". I never laughed outside of this group. People outside this group saw no humor. We also cried together, if someone had a reoccurrence.

Other sources of support were my two friends who made me prayer shawls: one to take to my chemo treatments and one to take to my radiation treatments; my girlfriend who took me to all of my treatments, and my wonderful husband, Miguel. He was very supportive and wanted to do as much as he could for me, without babying me, which was important. I knew, however, I needed to keep some normalcy in his life so I told him to go to work and allow my girlfriend and others to help out. Above all, God got me through every step of the way. My faith was a very important piece for me.

What used to stress me doesn't anymore. I look at life differently – my perspective has changed. What is now important is family, health, happiness and the ability to work. I am grateful that God has blessed me with the ability to work again.

Never having gone through anything like this before, myself or with someone else, I had a fear of the unknown. What was chemo like? I was clueless. I wish I had known more about possible side-effects and had better dietary instructions. It would have been nice to have the opportunity to sit down with a coach or counselor. Understandably, nurses don't have time. Although I wasn't brave enough to have all the facts put on the table and I'd shut down rather than ask the questions that I should have, I now realize the truth to Dr. Oz's line, "knowledge is power."

My experience with breast cancer has made me a better nurse. I am more empathetic and compassionate. Laying there on that bed not knowing what's going to happen scares you to death. Just talking to people helps them so much. I encourage patients and I ask if they have a caretaker and a support group.

I have learned that something good always comes out of something bad. I have met the most wonderful people through this experience that I wouldn't have met otherwise. I am now a sister and I really understand what it means.

Jo Rivera
As written by Diane Weller
(Family story of Vicki Kovatto, Jo Rivera, Miguel Rivera, Alexis Pino, and Michael Pino)

Jo and Miguel (next story) live in Reading, PA. Jo has been a nurse for 28 years and Miguel is retired. Miguel has five sons and one grandson. He enjoys music, reading, exercising, and retirement! Jo is active in the church, knits, reads, shops (loves to shop) and is currently pursuing her BSN. They have two cats and enjoy spending time with family.

A Pink Ribbon Story
Miguel Rivera

It's pretty scary, as a caretaker, to go through this with your wife. The news is devastating. It's a very tough situation, but I thank God for getting us through it.

I've never formulated my thoughts about having had this experience. But I know faith is big, because you feel like you are in a losing battle.

I never saw a stronger human being than my wife when she went through the procedures she did. She never once complained. It takes a special kind of person to go through this and not complain.

Her incredible strength and the fortitude she displayed helped me to be stronger. Still, some things are out of our control and we feel powerless. I tried not to show my feelings of being overwhelmed and the inward battles I was going through, but it was tough!

The experience brings your relationship even closer because there is something smack in the middle of you and you're fighting to become closer. There is always a positive to everything negative, if you take the time to look for it.

I would tell other caretakers to keep God in the picture. Your devotion to Him and constant prayer for help is a good way to get through. Without it, I don't know how we would have gotten through it.

During our experience I could find no humor in it and even looking back now, I see no humor in it. I guess this is in my roots from my father. To my father, a serious matter was taken seriously and no other way.

Miguel Rivera
As written by Diane Weller
(Family story of Vicki Kovatto, Jo Rivera, Miguel Rivera, Alexis Pino, and Michael Pino)

My Choice
Christine Rudy

During my very first oncologist appointment, one of the things my doctor said to me was that someday in some way, something good will come from this. I have to tell you, I thought he was crazy. My response to him as I sat in the office seven months ago was silence, but the whole time I was thinking: "Are you kidding me, how could anything good come from me being diagnosed with breast cancer?"

In the beginning I was terrified. Not so much for me, but for my family. I would lay awake at night thinking about my girls and worry that I wouldn't be able to spend the same amount of quality time with them as I did before I got sick. I would worry about them being able to deal with the issue emotionally. Most adults don't know how to deal with cancer, so how can we expect children to be able to deal with it? I felt horrible that my family would have to go through this. I have a wonderful husband and two beautiful daughters whose lives I knew were about to be turned upside down. I was right; the next several months were anything but "normal" for us. There were a lot of ups and downs, good days and not so good days.

When you are facing a difficult time in your life, you soon come to realize that you can't do everything yourself anymore and you need to rely on others. When you open yourself up to accept help, you learn a lot about people. How kind they can be, how helpful and encouraging they can be and how much people really want to help each other.

Some of the greatest forms of encouragement may come from old friends you haven't spoken with in years or people that you have only come to know because of your diagnosis. Two breast cancer survivors visited me at my home. They didn't know anything about me, but they openly shared their stories and experiences with me. Seeing these women and how well they were doing was a true inspiration to me.

314

I also realized a lot about myself. I began to view each day as a blessing and not worry about things I had no control over. I realized that the stuff that used to upset me in most cases wasn't that important and instead of getting upset, I tried to be more understanding and patient. I realized that I had the power within me, and through the support of my family and friends, to be courageous, to be strong, to be a survivor.

I truly believe that when it comes to cancer, attitude really is everything. My favorite quote of all time is "Life is 10% what happens to you and 90% how you react to it" – Charles R. Swindoll. Every situation gives us an opportunity to choose how we are going to react. I can choose to get consumed in the negativity that all too often accompanies cancer, or I can choose to look beyond the negativity, and realize all that I have been blessed with. I choose to recognize my blessings and be grateful for them. I choose to slow down and enjoy life. I choose to laugh every day and I choose to never give up and will "fight the fight."

I guess my oncologist was right after all. A short seven months later and I can already say that something good has come from this. I have witnessed the beautiful, kind and selfless side of so many people and have been reminded that other than a few disappointments, people truly are good, caring and compassionate. I have been reminded of who I am, what really matters to me and that I already have everything and more than I could possibly need in life.

Experiences that I could have only had due to cancer have created memories that I will cherish for the rest of my life: like the haircuts my daughter, Alli, gave me to help prepare me for my change in appearance; the day my daughters and their friends dyed pink streaks in their hair in support of me; the note of encouragement my husband wrote to me on my first day of chemo; when my daughter Carlee kissed me on the forehead and told me that I was still beautiful on the first day I was officially bald.

I have never once questioned "why me?" Instead I choose to focus on enjoying each moment of every day and trying to be the best wife, mom, sister, friend, and overall person I can be. Each day is a gift – I choose to enjoy it!

Christine resides in Mifflinburg, PA with her husband Wade and two daughters, Carlee and Alli. She enjoys spending quality time with family and friends, art and the outdoors. She is employed by Keystone Insurers Group in Northumberland, PA and can be contacted at therudys@windstream.net.

My Humble Opinion
Kathy Salloum

Tammy asked me to offer a few words about my experience as a Pink Ribbon Writer for this book. I would like to offer a special thank you to Tammy Miller and the other Pink Ribbon Story author's. It was an honor to work with the true hero's of life.

The opportunity to talk with some of the people whose stories are featured in this beautiful book has been a humbling and great experience.

"Attitude is a little thing that makes a big difference" (Winston Churchill) and these stories are a daily inspiration. So many of the stories are indicators of exactly what Churchill was referring to with this quote, and their attitude to overcome the difficult challenges of a breast cancer diagnosis is inspiring.

Thank you for the opportunity to be inspired by you!

A note of gratitude to Tavrie for her support and guidance.

Kathy Salloum was born in Edmonton, Alberta, and currently lives in State College, PA. She thanks God, parents Bud and Laverna Salloum, children Sean and Tavrie and Noelle...family and dear friends for her daily inspiration.

A Sprinkle of FUN from Tammy...

"A woman knows all about her children. She knows about dentist appointments, soccer games, romances, best friends, location of friend's houses, favorite foods, secret fears and hopes and dreams. A man is vaguely aware of some short people living in the house."

--Unknown

A Health Detective
Gloria Santiago

I was once asked, "Doesn't cancer suck?" I answered, "No, cancer changed my life. It changed my perspective on how I treat people. I no longer take people for granted. I have learned to be humble and grateful."

In fact, I would not be the Chief Detective in a Public Defender's Office had it not been for my journey through breast cancer. My 'detective' work all started in the spring of 2000. During a routine monthly self-breast exam, I found a lump on my left breast that wasn't there before. The doctor I worked for told me there was nothing to worry about. Six years later, I decided to investigate matters myself, asked questions and scheduled tests.

Days seem like years when you are waiting for test results. I finally scheduled an appointment with the surgeon myself, and the results: carcinoma. I have always had God in my life, but after hearing the diagnosis…it was time to fully embrace my faith. Growing up, I used to ask God to remove mountains. Now I just ask him to help me walk through them.

My faith had already seen me through 20 surgeries that made up my life's history this far. Before the next appointment with the surgeon, I found a lump on my right breast. A bilateral mastectomy was then scheduled.

I have always been a strong person, and comforted everyone else in time of need. My family and friends were so worried; they treated me like I was disabled. My father would bring me my coffee. When I told him my legs worked perfectly and I could get the coffee myself, it's like he didn't hear. Another valuable lesson…accept help from others! From the moment I was diagnosed, my father was there for me. My biological father was there for me too, but my "step" Dad took care of me every step of the way.

After my bilateral mastectomy, I returned to the cancer center and they told me there was no trace of cancer, but had to take Tamoxifin as follow up. My body had adverse reactions.

Even the blankets hurt. After a week and a half, I stopped the treatment.

In September 2006, my lymph nodes started to swell. Pathology came up fine, but I knew something wasn't quite right. A week later, I started feeling bumps on my spine. I rapidly deteriorated to the point that I had trouble moving my legs and hips. I was eventually life - flighted to the Cleveland Hospital and endured 2 months of bone scans and tests. It turns out I had a degenerative disease.

But all was not lost. When my former co-workers, family, and friends found out about my disease, everyone rallied. They organized fundraisers to help me pay my medical bills. Before my husband left me, he wanted me to have breast reconstruction. (I was just hoping to live until Christmas) After the separation, I decided to get reconstruction done. Two days after my expanders were put in place, I lost all feeling from the waist down. Eight days later, the doctor found tumors on my femur. You can imagine my dismay when I was told I had to be in a wheelchair for the next year.

Instead of putting God to the test, I just asked for strength. When I had a follow-up MRI and X-RAY of the femur to check on the tumors 11 months later, the tumors were gone. There was once proof I had cancerous tumors…and now they were gone. Miracle from God? Absolutely.

My story is truly a blessing. For the months that followed, I struggled with months of rehabilitation, from wheelchair to walker, to cane. I returned to school, graduating in December 2010 with a Criminal Justice degree. While going to University I ended up with 5 more surgeries, including the removal of my gall bladder and pancreas. Dr. Ostrowski from Gannon University was my rock, and still is. He believed in me even when I had my doubts. I went on to receive a Master's Degree and am now the Chief Detective in the Public Defenders Office in Erie, Pennsylvania. Who knew my real life detective skills during my breast cancer journey would not only save my life, but would also give me determination, dedication, a career and a life I love.

Words of advice? Be proactive with your health.   Take care of yourself. Be your own health detective. And above all else - believe.

Gloria Santiago
As written by Kathy Salloum

A Sprinkle of FUN from Tammy…

I hate housework. You make the beds, you wash the dishes and six months later you have to start all over again.

(It states that this is of "unknown" origin, but I think I should just put my name here as the Author – it works for me!!!)

-- Unknown??

I'm Not in Denial
Cheryl Saul

My life has been met with some pretty tough challenges, but the one I have embarked now has been my toughest.

Back in 1983 when a speeding drunk driver ran a stop sign and broadsided us, my body had its share of turmoil. Between surgery, seizures and a diagnosis of Syringomyelia (a cyst that planted itself inside my spinal cord and remains there), I learned to adapt and push my body beyond what the specialists thought I should do.

In the fall of '04 I was told I had suspicious nodules on my thyroid. While my family doctor was concerned and sent me for tests, a specialist and surgeon at the time dismissed it as nothing. I would have pursued it but a family crisis and death caused me to put it on the back burner. Fast forward to '08 when I could feel the one nodule, so I continued the pursuit for clear answers. After grueling months of biopsies that kept coming back inconclusive, the oncology surgeon decided it was time to remove half or all of the thyroid and then get a clearer pathology report. Surgery was done October 2009 and it came back not cancer. What a relief…or so I thought.

I had some joy about the results briefly, then the worry set right back in to my brain that something wasn't right. It was like I had a little person sitting on my shoulder whispering, "keep looking, you're not done yet." Two weeks into my recuperation I felt a sharp burning pain to the left side of my left breast. The area remained tender to the touch, like skin would feel if burned. Imagine my surprise to feel a lump. I already had a doctor appointment set up for thyroid level check within the week so I addressed the lump at that time and she was concerned, but said it could be just a cyst. A diagnostic mammogram was set for November 20th.

On November 19, 2009, I was feeling pretty confident that the results would show a cyst when I had examined myself again and thought the lump was smaller. I was wrong.

The diagnostic mammogram was awfully uncomfortable and extra views were taken. I was whisked off to ultrasound, and could read the radiologist's thoughts and expressions like an open book. They needed to do an immediate biopsy. There seems to be a sense of urgency here! I am at the hospital all alone and they are telling me I have cancer? My whole system went into shock. I remember two nurses gently walking me to a room, bundling me up in warm blankets and helping me call my husband at work. They wanted him to come, but I wanted to be the one to talk to him on the phone. I could hear his whole world of hopes and dreams dissolve right over the phone when I heard his cry as he was hanging up the phone. I later learned from his staff that he nearly collapsed in grief.

My husband arrived thankfully before I was taken away for the biopsies. We needed alone time. We had just enough alone time before I was shipped off to a room with more strange medical equipment. I am not going to go into all of the details as it sounds so frightening, but in the end it was okay.

The day before Thanksgiving, I put myself in "holiday mode" so that I wouldn't be thinking about the "C" word. The news wasn't good. The doctor explained it was infiltrating ductal carcinoma (invasive breast cancer) and possible lymph node involvement. I would need a surgeon for mastectomy and an oncologist for treatment. Happy Thanksgiving, huh?

I had my appointment with my surgeon to discuss my options. The PET scan revealed the cancer as 2cm, possible stage 2, high grade and triple negative. I will be having chemotherapy first, he says. It helps reduce the size of the tumor prior to surgery to make reconstruction easier, and chemo helps kill off anything hiding elsewhere. This approach is called neo-adjuvant therapy – chemo BEFORE surgery.

My first infusion was four days before Christmas. By New Year's my hair had begun to fall out. The hair follicles hurt so much that one day before my husband got home, I buzzed the rest of my hair off with his razor. As soon as he came home, we both laughed until we cried. He said he was very proud of me. I chose to wear a wig to spare my family members the sight of me looking ill. The image of my brother-in-law's bald, gaunt look through his cancer journey and then his death was still too fresh on their minds and I didn't want to be compared nor have them think that I would die too. The wig was comfortable but I had to go through the last half of cancer treatment during the hottest summer on record. I still continued to wear the wig through the summer until we attended a Phillies baseball game in 98 degree heat. By the 5th inning I needed to swap the wig for a light bucket hat I packed in my bag. I was getting light-headed and overheated. I made a mad dash for the ladies' room and was surprised to find myself alone. This is a rarity at a sporting event. I decided to take advantage of this by sticking my bald head under some cool water of the faucet. Out of the corner of my eye I caught a glimpse of a young girl who took one look at me and must have thought she had mistakenly entered the men's room. She turned and high-tailed it out of the rest room. I felt bad for her but I couldn't help but find the humor in my situation.

I didn't know that the combination of chemo drugs and the steroids used to combat chemo reactions would cause weight gain. I didn't just gain a few pounds, I gained a lot! To cope with the shock of my diagnosis, wintry blues and isolation from germs and bacteria, I began to search for online breast cancer support groups, blogs and networks, as well as keep family and friends up to date on my progress via a Facebook note page. I refused to let fear and depression set in.

Surprisingly, the time flew by quickly and the last chemo was in sight. New tests performed before surgery showed that my 2cm tumor was gone! Chemo had done its job. I changed my mind about a full mastectomy and chose a lumpectomy instead. Sentinel node biopsy showed no lymph node involvement. I began radiation one month after surgery and was given 35 doses. Everything went well until the last week when I suffered a nasty and painful burn near the neck/clavicle area. It was quite large in circumference, deep, and frightening to look at. In a Zumba class shortly thereafter, I wore a gauze bandage around my neck to hold the burn dressings and so no one would gawk at my wound. After about 15 minutes of Zumba, my dressings slid away from the burn and my Aunt had a look of panic. There I was looking like someone had try to decapitate me. The following class had my husband and my Aunt encouraging me to ditch the wig for comfort, so now I show up to the same class with no wig. I wonder what must have gone through those ladies' minds. First my "Frankenstein" neck, then my hair is missing. Oh the fun of trying to read their faces.

I have an occasional "chemo brain" moment, feel some neuropathy come and go, but for the most part I feel my body slowly returning to a better state. I am finding my new normal. It's apparent the old normal is gone. Every little ache or pain brings the fear of the unknown. I am blessed to have a superb caregiver, my husband, who never faltered in his loving support. According to Marc Silver, author of the "Breast Cancer Husband," my husband learned the best thing he could do was "shut up and listen." When he told me I was beautiful whether I had hair or not, I knew he was the 'wind beneath my wings.' The man is incredible. Crazy as this sounds, I had asked him to purchase a puppy for me shortly after my first chemo infusion, and with a little hesitation he did so. A sweet little puppy graced my feel bad days with warm kisses, puppy breath, and yes…piddle puddles, but I had something to focus on besides throwing myself a pity party. Little Baxter's one-year birthday and Thanksgiving fall right at the time of my diagnosis the year before. They will both be a reason to celebrate thankfulness of life.

My biggest lesson is to find something to laugh at every day. There's nothing wrong with a cancer patient having humor! Some people mistake humor as denial. Laughing is not only good for the soul, but it's good for the body too. I'm grateful for my supportive husband, daughter, family, friends, and of course Baxter.

Cheryl Saul lives in Emmaus, PA. with her husband and dog, Baxter. She is a mother of one daughter and Nanni to a beautiful granddaughter. She enjoys gardening, cross-stitching, traveling and spending time with family. She is currently active in raising money for cancer research.

A Sprinkle of FUN from Tammy...

"Any mother could perform the jobs of several air-traffic controllers with ease."   -- Lisa Alther

Upstairs, Downstairs
Shelby Shoemaker

I was no stranger to cancer. My parents died from cancer. My mother died at 36 years of age from colon cancer. My father died at 46 years of age from lung cancer. I felt as though I was predisposed to cancer. In 1989 I was diagnosed with colon cancer. I thought it was a death sentence. Through surgery, exercise and healthful living, I found the diagnosis was, in fact, not a death sentence. In 2002, I was diagnosed with breast cancer. I realized it was time to arm myself with knowledge and prepare once again for battle with cancer.

Shortly after diagnosis many things became a blur. Some became quite clear. If you don't have your health, you don't have anything. It is amazing how something like this can put your entire life in perspective. It makes you aware of how much the little things matter. Your thought process changes as does your outlook on life. Every single day is a blessing.

My husband, three children, grandchildren and daughters in - law were very supportive. I knew I was blessed when my husband said, "I love you, not your boobs." My daughter happily told me that now my boobs can be whatever size I want, and I won't sag when I get old. My boobs can be "up" and perky forever. Hair grows back and boobs come in all sizes. My church family was over the top. So is the power of prayer.

The initial diagnosis of cancer can be a shock…but know it can change things for the better in every way. This does not mean to ignore what you are feeling. Go through the stages, the anger, fear and denial. Be honest and truthful with yourself. Give yourself permission to feel. When you have to wait for results, you're going to be scared, no matter what! Breast cancer is an extremely personal disease. No one can really prepare you for your journey, but know you are not alone. Your support groups can help share your struggles and celebrate your victories.

When I was diagnosed, I felt like I had joined a club I did not want to belong to. I decided to start a club, a support group, I really wanted to belong to. That group, "Pink Ribbon Girls", started with 4 ladies and now we are 31 members strong. Being a part of a group doesn't necessarily mean you have to plan agendas and "minutes." Sometimes all we did was hug and cry.

In May of 2002, my son's Mother and Father - in - law, Ruth and Jim Jackson, formed a Relay For Life team in my honor called "One Step At A Time." This angel team of 30 members, raised more than $130,000.00 over the course of eight years for breast cancer research. The research that helps us get one step closer to discovering better medications and ultimately finding a cure for this disease.

I have been blessed with early detection in both cases. My colonoscopy in 1989 and mammogram in 2002 saved my life. Early detection is SO important. Become your own patient advocate. Ask questions, and then ask more questions. Write your questions down for the next visit. If you do not have good rapport with your surgeon or oncologist, find another doctor. Learn about your options. Take care of yourself. Support the American Cancer Society. If it were not for the latest research and the newest medications, my story may have been a bit different. Being a survivor is a gift. Offering support is a gift you can give back.

As for the title....... Humor plays a big role in breast cancer recovery. One morning my husband came downstairs and said "Wow! You are down stairs!" I questioned with "Where did you think I was?" He replied "Well, I wasn't sure. Your boobs are up here."

Shelby Shoemaker
As written by Kathy Salloum

Shelby is the mother of three children, five grand children, and one great grandson. She has been happily married for 50 years. She and is a registered nurse after graduating from Polyclinic Hospital in Harrisburg, PA in 1961. She started a breast cancer support group 5 years ago called Pink Ribbon Girls and any girls who have cancer are welcome to join the group. They meet once a month and have a great time sharing and laughing together. Her number is 814-643-3254, please call if she can be of any support to anyone.

A Sprinkle of FUN from Tammy...

"Adam and Eve had an ideal marriage. He didn't have to hear about all the men she could have married, and she didn't have to hear about the way his mother cooked."

--Kimberly Broyles

Wings, Anchors and Life Preservers
Karen Shuman

WINGS, ANCHORS AND LIFE PRESERVERS.............
My reaction to my diagnosis was probably typical of most: shock, fear and "let's get moving on this". I do believe that several factors fell into place for me, helping to achieve a positive outcome. These factors I refer to (lovingly, of course) are my WINGS, ANCHORS and LIFE PRESERVERS. Without hesitation, my family, friends and co-workers stepped up to fill these roles.

FIRST AND FOREMOST.... MY WINGS.........
Before speaking to my kids about my diagnosis, my best friend, Deb cried with me, comforted my heart and prayed with me. Then she arranged the most wonderful gift, a meeting with her pastor. Just the three of us prayed, an anointing with oil and an offering of a comfort zone from which to operate was given to me. When I couldn't lift my heart and soul because of the fear, Deb and Pastor Marlys graciously lent their wings to help my fearful ones to fly. A wonderful sense of calm and hope helped me to focus during the difficult times. This was my gift for which I am daily grateful.

My BFF since childhood, Barb was only a phone call away. I wrote a long, gut wrenching letter to Barb about my diagnosis asking her to be with me if needed. Somehow, writing those words down on paper helped me to "own" my diagnosis of cancer. Barb has always been my "wingman" for any difficulties in life and this was no different. You see, she is a cancer survivor herself and knew exactly where my heart and head were not very far off the ground. Many times and at inconvenient hours, I would call and just let it all pour out. Barb has always possessed strong and loving wings. Without missing a beat, she managed to keep me airborne during the rough days of chemo, impending surgery and radiation. Lots of times, I did a crash and burn, dangerously close to ending it all. Barb was there and pulled me upward.

And then there's Luann, not only a best friend and confidant, but my teacher assistant and an excellent one at that. I know I was in her prayers daily and her words of encouragement and cards were gratefully accepted and appreciated. "Gee, you look great" kept me buoyant and positive because most of the time I certainly didn't feel that way. I rarely shared my struggles at work, but Luann knew what I was feeling and with her strength kept me hovering. We often teased that when we retire from teaching, we're heading on a "girls only cruise". It may just happen! To this day one of the cards she sent me remains and will remain on my kitchen corkboard. The card reads, "You are stronger than you realize." It's a daily reminder and a good one for any of us. My life, my soul, and my future I owe to my WINGS.

SECOND, THOSE SOLID ANCHORS........
The anchors in my life are obvious choices, my children and my brother. Believe it or not, it was most difficult for me to tell my brother of my diagnosis and I avoided it for a while. You see, just thirty short years before we had lost our Mom to cancer and my kid brother, Bill was stunned, but supportive. He and his wife, Mary offered to fly in and be there for me which, I am most grateful. My kids, my babies, my pride and joy, my frustrating moments of parenting, my heart and soul and my reason for living are in Josh, Seth, Noah and Sarah Kate and a lovely daughter in law, Jess. In their handsome, gorgeous and intelligent faces I see the best of gifts; the best of me and the worst of me, the future, great promise and potential and I was selfish enough to want to experience it all for myself. When I was hooked up to chemo or "my chemical romance" as I called it, it was those faces I focused on when I drifted off to my zone of comfort and just meditated. For them, I fought. My anchors kept me tethered to this planet when it would have been easiest just to drift away.

LASTLY AND MOST IMPORTANTLY..........LIFE PERESERVERS.......

After my youngest son benefitted from wonderful care at University of Pittsburgh Medical Center, I decided if I ever needed care I would head to Magee Women's Hospital. Their exemplary knowledge, care and compassion is the best medicine anyone can hope for. My team treated my diagnosis, but cared for the person. When I was frightened (which was most of the time) there was a hand in mine or someone next to me; when I cried there was a compassionate heart sitting next to me and when I was silent there was someone nearby checking on me. Once again, I must reiterate, Magee Women's Hospital and Women's Cancer Center have exemplary knowledge, exemplary care and exemplary compassion to offer. Three cheers for Dr. Rastogi and her wonderful "crew'. Three cheers for LIFE PRESERVERS.

Every morning when I wake up, often during the day and in the closing hours of my day, I repeat two small, but heartfelt words, "Thank you" aimed heaven ward . For without my WINGS, ANCHORS and LIFE PRESERVERS I would have crashed to Earth so many times. My second grandson, Isaac was born the morning I began my chemicals. As his NANA, I just can't get enough of his hugs and smiles. His name means "he who laughs or brings laughter". I plan on doing just that: laughing with my kids, my grandbabies, my friends and with life!

Karen Shuman
Ivan and Bettie's only daughter, a sister, a Mom, a teacher, a best friend, a survivor ………………

Karen lives quite contentedly in Hollidaysburg,PA. Having taken the "road less travelled" has made all the difference in her personal and professional life. She can be reached at: Isaacsnana52@Yahoo.com

My Dealing With Cancer
Jan Siberine

One thing that I found extremely helpful while going through treatment was a book called Dr. Susan Love's Breast Book. To me, it is more or less the bible for women affected by breast cancer. It was brought to my attention by a neighbor, and from then on, I used it as a daily guide. It describes breast development and physiology, appearance and common noncancerous conditions as well as breast cancer in a wise and warm fashion. It assisted me through the steps of everything I encountered along the way. I was also put in contact with my friend's cousin who had the exact type of cancer that I had, and had gone through all of the same surgeries I was facing. This was extremely beneficial because she was able to give me a heads-up about what each surgery would entail, and what side effects I should expect. She made it much easier for me because I wasn't going into any of the procedures blind.

The support of other cancer patients is something that has been very special to me; it's like an unspoken bond that you form, knowing that these women have gone through the same thing that you are going through. There is an incredible organization near my house called The Wellness Center. They offer yoga classes and support groups free of charge for women who are survivors. Whenever I'm having a bad day, I know I can go there and surround myself with others who can easily relate to my situation. If I go to a support meeting, I don't even have to talk. Rather, I can just sit and listen to others tell their stories, which is something I find great comfort in.

Jan Siberine
As written by Kelsey Itak
Jan lives in Hillsborough, N.J. She was diagnosed with breast cancer at the age of 49. She had a Mastectomy and reconstruction surgery and is currently taking Tamoxifen. She continues to keep a positive attitude on her life and gives emotional support to anyone who needs it.

The Beginning of a New Me
Kalpa Solanski

It was June, 2007 - my birthday month. I was turning 40 and looking forward to it. After all, the 40s were supposed to be the new 30s. Not sure what that means, but Oprah says it, so it must be true! I was hoping that this decade of my life would be full of confidence and self assurance, wisdom and new-found appreciation for who I am.

I take pretty good care of myself. I eat relatively healthy, exercise sporadically, and maintain a generally healthy lifestyle. I may not be consistent with taking the vitamins or meds that are prescribed to me...but I know that it is important to see my internist, gynecologist, and eye doctor for routine visits. So when I received the script for my 40-year-old mammogram, I approached it as a rite of passage into my fourth decade of life. Little did I know that it was going to be the beginning of a "new" me.

It was just days after my birthday that I was given my diagnosis of high grade DCIS (ductal carcinoma in situ), and it was overwhelming and surreal at the same time. The hardest thing for me to comprehend was how I could be sick and not even feel sick? I didn't have any risk factors except that I had breasts. I am relatively young and in decent shape. I don't smoke and only drink socially. I don't have a family history of breast cancer, and I am of an ethnicity that is usually at lower risk. So Why Me? Then I realized that I am no more special than anyone else who got cancer so Why Not Me?

The diagnosis of cancer changes you forever. I spent many days and nights crying and being scared for my life. In fact, there are days that I still cry, but they are now few and far between. No matter how much information you have about your diagnosis, cancer in any form seems like a death sentence. I discovered that in a way it was...a death sentence. It was the death of the "old me."

With that said, breast cancer has opened opportunities for me I never would have expected. Those hopes of confidence, self assurance, wisdom, and self appreciation I longed for... breast cancer gave them to me.

I am an occupational therapist by education. I graduated from Thomas Jefferson University with a Bachelor's and Master's degree in Occupational Therapy. I worked in my field for 12 years before "retiring" to raise my kids. Ironically, 15 years ago, I completed my Master's thesis on "Role Changes following a Mastectomy" and also developed an exercise and lymphedema program for the hospital I was affiliated with at the time. Never did I think that I would come to rely on that information for my own recovery.

However, as I was undergoing my surgical treatment, I was *underwhelmed* by the information, or lack of information, given to me regarding my recovery process. Subsequent to my diagnosis, two of my dear friends were diagnosed with the disease and came to me for support and advice. I realized then that I had valuable and practical information to share. I was encouraged by my husband to put my information down on paper, and that is how I came to write **The Mastectomy Manual**.

The manual is a compilation of my research, feedback from other breast cancer patients, and more importantly, my own experience as a patient and therapist. I also used my education and work experience to develop a breast cancer rehab program to help women restore function following their breast surgery.

Three years following my initial diagnosis, I received another scare. During my mammogram of my remaining breast, there was a suspicious mass discovered. Fortunately for me, the mass was benign. However, after careful consideration, my husband and I made a decision to remove that breast as well. I no longer have my original breasts and my body has been slightly altered, but I thank God everyday for taking me on this journey. I know now that I am stronger than any problem I encounter or any disappointment that life will bring. I am stronger than I ever knew.

Kalpa Solanki
As written by Kelsey Itak

Kalpa Solanki lives in Sinking Spring, PA with her husband Raj and 2 children. She is an occupational therapist and the founder of Comprehensive Breast Cancer Rehabilitation at The Berks Hand Therapy Center in Wyomissing, PA. She can be reached at www.mastectomyexercises.com.

A Sprinkle of FUN from Tammy…

"Cleaning your house while your kids are still growing is like shoveling the walk before it stops snowing."   ---Phyllis Diller

I'm Not Cousin Hattie
Joyce Sprague

The first person I knew who had breast cancer was my mother's first cousin, Hattie. It was late afternoon in 1970 when I walked into my grandmother's living room just in time to witness a whispered conversation between my mother, my grandmother, and a teary-eyed Cousin Hattie. I was only seventeen years old but I immediately knew something was seriously wrong when my mother shooed me out of the room without explanation. Indeed, something was wrong. But when I was growing up in North Carolina no one I knew uttered the words "breast cancer." It may have been because Southern polite society did not mention women's body parts as much as it was the fear of the disease itself. Within two years Hattie was dead. It was not until May 1989 that I heard the words "breast cancer" again, one week after my 37th birthday. This time, however, the words were about me, and they changed my life forever.

Inflammatory Breast Cancer (IBC) is rare and very aggressive. It can cause redness, swelling, and warmth in the breast, but it does not always have a distinct lump. In fact, one doctor treated me with antibiotics for several weeks because he thought I had mastitis (inflammation of the breast). Unfortunately, IBC does not show up on a mammogram and often spreads before it is diagnosed, one reason for its low 5-year survival rate of 25% – 50%.

At the time of my diagnosis, my primary surgeon asked me to trust him and told me that we would take it one day at a time. My second-opinion surgeon told me that I had three months to live because, based on preliminary tests, the cancer had spread throughout my body. I gave up hope! After leaving his office, I began to mentally give away my possessions. Even when a voice spoke to me while on my way home in the car telling me, "You're going to be all right," I thought my husband, who was driving, had spoken to me or that I was hallucinating. Because of my Christian faith, I wasn't afraid to die, but I was afraid that I would not live to see our two daughters graduate from high school (Kimberly was 12 years old and Shannon 15). I was afraid of leaving my family and friends, and most of all, I was afraid of leaving the girls in the care of a man who was not a good father to them. He loved me but never wanted kids so, at the time, pretty much ignored them.

Kim, who would drag her bedding into the living room because she didn't want me to be alone as I vomited for most of the night after a session of chemotherapy, told me she thought I was courageous. I've never considered myself courageous. I just did what I had to do. When my second-opinion surgeon told me that I had three months to live, I could have chosen to curl up into a fetal position and wait for death to come, or I could have chosen to live. I admit that it took me a few days, but I finally made the choice to live. One day at a time. None of us is promised tomorrow, but we can choose not to die mentally, emotionally, and spiritually while waiting for our physical death.

I chose to go through the industrial-strength chemotherapy and the radiation that followed because I had hope. Hope that the treatments would work and, if they didn't, that the doctors could keep me alive long enough for the scientists to find something that would. I knew that my God did not deal in statistics so I quit reading books that told me what the odds were that I would die. Because I wanted to help in some way with my recovery, I began practicing visualization. At first, as I lay on the couch with my eyes closed, I imagined a huge elephant vacuuming up cancer seeds with his trunk, but I hate housework so quickly abandoned the image. Next, I imagined a Gatlin gun blasting cancerous boulders, but I found the image too violent. My third attempt pictured a dozen small doves eating cancer seeds at the bottom of a turreted tower. Once they gorged themselves, they flew away. I was able to recall the image multiple times but gradually summoned fewer and fewer doves until finally only one large dove materialized. He never descended to the now barren floor. He quietly gazed at me from the open window and then he was gone. I was never able to imagine the doves again, but I felt in my spirit that the cancer was gone.

My oncologist once called me his star patient, and maybe I am because I survived IBC, but he will also tell you that I was a basket case during my recovery. In fact, God might also tell you that I was a basket case because, although I was practically reared in the church by Christian parents, He heard more from me during that period of my life than He had in years. Of course, there was an outpouring of support from my family and friends, and especially from my husband who held me at night when I cried, and who told me that he didn't marry me for my body parts so it was all right that I only had one breast. He kept his cool when he told me gently that I was going to be o.k. and I snapped back at him because, as I told him, "You aren't God! How do you know everything is going to be o.k."! And he loved me anyway. Sometimes I think it is harder on our family and friends than it is on those of us who are going through it. I hope that I always remember to say thank you to anyone who is or who has ever been a caregiver because I am not the only survivor in the battle against breast cancer. They are survivors, too.

I don't take survivorship for granted because my survival made it possible for me to see both of our daughters not only graduate from high school but graduate from college and then marry. It allowed me to continue to work full-time at Gettysburg College while also taking classes part-time, graduating Phi Beta Kappa in 2003 (at the age of 51) with a BA in Classical Studies and a minor in Religion. I also had the privilege many years ago of becoming a Reach to Recovery volunteer for the American Cancer Society. Because a Reach to Recovery volunteer, Twila Charles, once gave me encouragement and hope, I want to support other women diagnosed with breast cancer. When I first met Twila, she complained that she really needed a haircut now that her hair had grown back (and I knew that in a few short weeks I would be bald), and she was on her way to go waterskiing (something that I used to do). I remember staring in amazement as she drove out of my driveway. It was then that I realized that there IS life after breast cancer.

Joyce, a transplanted North Carolinian, lives in Orrtanna, PA with Walt, her loving husband of 41 years, and their two cats, Apollo and Athena. She is the Academic Administrative Assistant for the Women, Gender, and Sexuality Studies Program at Gettysburg College. You can reach her at jsprague@gettysburg.edu.

A Sprinkle of FUN from Tammy...

"Life was so much easier when your clothes didn't match and boys had cooties!"   --Unknown

A Telephone Call One Never Expects!
Lisa Spuhler

A telephone call one never expects or wants to receive –
"your mammogram showed some 'abnormal' calcium deposits and
we need to perform another mammogram". Being divorced, I
choose to walk into the doctor's office for my follow-up
mammogram and to hear the results with my Higher Power. After
receiving the recommendation to have a biopsy performed and
selecting my best friend's breast cancer surgeon, I know my
Higher Power carried me out of that office.

I feel very blessed that we caught the abnormal calcium
deposits very early. I was always faithful to myself by having my
annual mammograms as every woman should do for herself. The
cancer center staff said, I was "a candidate for a billboard to help
educate other women". It turned out; I had Ductal Carcinoma In
Situ (DCIS). DCIS is not invasive and could be removed by a
lumpectomy. Having no experience with breast cancer and my
head spinning, I trusted and followed my doctor's
recommendations. I decided to stay off of the internet reading
information that would scare and confuse me. I needed to keep my
survival attitude to reassure my daughter who was petrified that
she was going to lose me. Her support and love was just the
prescription I needed to persevere.

Round two of another lumpectomy was needed due to the
margins being too close (there wasn't enough healthy tissue around
the site). I almost passed out during the "needle" location. They
perform a mammogram to insert a hooked needle at the site to
guide the surgeon. They needed to move the needle while I was
still clamped down in the mammogram machine. Before I knew it
they had me out of the machine, laid back and my feet up in the
air. When I got color back in my face, the doctor called me a
"wimp" – "damn right I am…."!

Once I recovered from the surgeries, the next step was 33
treatments of radiation. I was in a panic for a few days of my
treatment as the nurse instructed me not to wear deodorant for my

treatments and I wasn't scheduled until 3:30 PM. How could I possibly work all day with NO deodorant and NOT smell? Turns out, I couldn't apply deodorant an "hour" before my treatment so applying it in the morning was just fine – maybe I missed that part of the instructions? I won't even mention the lengths I went to not stink all day at work – like putting a panty shield in the arm pit of my tops to absorb the sweat....

As I was leaving work for my first radiation treatment, a co-worker didn't have a clue where I was going but said to me "knock-um dead". I laughed as I walked to my car because that was exactly what I was hoping we'd do! My co-workers played a big part of me getting through the entire process with their love and support. It was amazing how we women bonded while waiting for our radiation treatments every Monday through Friday. Flannel gowns would have been nice for us cold blooded people. As the weeks progressed, I realized how special the technicians were by their caring nature and fun loving characters. They gave us all a sense that we were just fine and made our last treatment like a graduation.

Be prepared to show your boobies to everyone! I MEAN EVERYONE - mammogram techs, surgeon, oncologist, radiologist, radiation techs – everyone gets to check um out!!!! And don't be surprised when you run into one of your "young good-looking male technicians" at a restaurant. When I saw him, all I could think about was "he has seen my boobs"! But, when we chatted, he was the wonderful sweet radiation tech that he always was during my treatments.

At first the medication, tamoxifen, was a challenge. After a few weeks of dealing with feeling inadequate at everything I did, my best friend happened to share that tamoxifen made her "dumb". I couldn't believe it – I was suffering from feeling "dumb" at work, at home – even getting words out properly was a challenge. I can't tell you how many times I walked out of my boss' office in tears due to forgetting something "again" or just doing things wrong "again". My co-workers were real troopers putting up with my dumbness and we choose to enjoy my silliness with laughter at the things I said and did. I visited the doctor and she prescribed Lexapro (anti-depressant) which helped level out the effects of the tamoxifen and I was back to normal in no time (well, if you ask my co-workers they might not describe me as "normal"). So, remember to share your experience with others because we can always help each other.

I spent eight great weeks attending a breast cancer class "Prescription for Life". The dedicated cancer center staff taught us that reducing our fat intake may help lessen our chances of reoccurrence. They inspired us to try new fat free foods, healthier recipes, and learn new ways to relax and exercise. The care the staff provided and up lifting attitudes reinforced a positive outlook in all of us women. During the class, I realized that not all surgeons instruct their patients to massage their incision to keep it from hardening. This was something I could share with other women – she recommended massaging for two years after surgery.

I recently met a really special person to share my life with and my lumpectomy doesn't make a difference in my physical appearance to him. He thinks I'm beautiful and treats both of my breasts in the same loving way….

In December 2010, I passed my one year checkup and look forward to passing every checkup in the future. I am so blessed!

Lisa lives in Manchester, PA. She has two children, a 25-year old son and a 19-year old daughter. Her son is married and they have blessed her with a lively 4-year old grandson. Lisa says her children, daughter-in-law, and grandson are what help keep her young and alive! She is an Office Manager for an accounting firm and can be reached at omispuhler@comcast.net.

Reaching the Light
Lael Swank

I was diagnosed with breast cancer at 39 years old. From the very beginning, I was extremely open about my disease, which ultimately led to the structuring of the most incredible support group I ever could have asked for. My best friend and motivator through everything, Linda, shared an analogy that has always been very special to me:

Since March, you found yourself in a basement "somewhere" with a backpack tossed on and you've been trying to get to a light up above you ever since. Each day, you climb a set of stairs in the hopes of one day reaching the top. Each day, the load you started with gets heavier. You wonder why and realize that your old life didn't disappear. It remains with you along with all the struggles each new day brings. Along the way you stop. You duck in the stairwell so no one will see and you try and catch your breath. After this respite you continue your steps having taken it all in again.

Another day arrives and the fog above clears a little and hope is again renewed. You look below and smile at how many stairs you have climbed. Weight has been removed from your shoulders and quicker steps immediately follow. But just as fast as this glimmer shines, smoke again forms in front of your eyes. Still continuing your quest, another day brings another flight of stairs. Your backpack slowly gets heavier again and you remember when there were days that seemed long ago when wearing one this heavy never occurred to you.

So many tomorrows have come and you've taken flight each time. Repeating your steps through struggles and triumphs all the while anticipating the day when you've reached the top and can exchange your backpack for a smaller size and never have to catch your breath in a stairwell again.

Amazingly enough, my "army" of support was with me from the first step. I was so fortunate to have my family, lifelong friends, and my community to help me during the climb. From babysitting my two sons to preparing meals, everyone was rallying for me. My husband, of course, was my biggest support. He drove me to Philadelphia for every appointment I had and provided me with the love I needed to help me heal. Another person who stepped up to the plate from Day One was Linda. She approached me about CarePages, an online blog, which she thought I should utilize to keep friends and family informed throughout the journey. She offered to post the photos and updates so that I wouldn't have to worry about keeping up with it every day; this was also beneficial because I didn't have to field frequent phone calls about how everything was going. Linda and I spoke on a regular basis – we would talk, cry, laugh, joke, and all the while, she was keeping a log in the back of her head to update my CarePages.

Another special person who helped me through my journey was my friend Jill. Just before I lost my hair, she made me a basket with hats, bandanas, makeup, fun earrings and jammies. This is one of the most emotional stages, especially for women, so I really appreciated her efforts to help me feel more feminine and beautiful.

One day, I was talking online with a close friend who had moved to Germany shortly after my diagnosis. It was one of those days when I had to stop to take a breath in the stairwell, and she could tell I was struggling. About 30 minutes later, my doorbell rang and I opened it to find another friend of mine with flowers, a box of tissues, and coffee. My friend in Germany had called her because she didn't want me to be alone when I was so upset. I was amazed that day to realize how many incredible people I had in my life. She helped me catch my breath; I stood back up, and continued up the stairs.

After four and a half months, I was finally done with all 16 chemotherapy treatments. On my way home from Fox Chase Cancer Center, there were pink streamers and balloons tied to trees along the half-mile route up to my house, which was decked out in just as much pink apparel. On my front step, there was also dinner prepared and waiting. It was truly remarkable. A neighbor who saw all of the decorated trees actually thought that I had just come home from having a baby, which gave everyone a good laugh. Later that night, my husband told me that our boys had a surprise for me outside. I walked out the garage to find about 75 of my friends and family walking down my street, all holding candles. They were there to celebrate my chemo graduation. Once again, I was taken back by how much love enveloped me, and my backpack began to feel lighter.

Just before I reached the light at the top of the stairs, all the students in my son Garrett's 3rd grade class made me cards out of construction paper. I visited the students to bring them lollipops, thank them for the cards, and show them I was doing well. One card in particular stood out to me. A little girl wrote, "Mrs. Swank, I think you are the only person I know who has cancer." This really struck me because, at such a young age, she was probably right – I most likely was the only person she knew who has had cancer. But since breast cancer affects 1 in 8 women, statistically, two girls in that class will grow up and be diagnosed with the disease. I am hopeful that, because I was so open about it, the hypothetical two that will eventually be diagnosed won't be as afraid. I hope that their interaction with me will provide them with courage, strength, and ultimately a much smaller backpack.

Lael Swank
As written by Kelsey Itak

Lael lives in Mountain Top, PA with her husband, Randy, and two sons, Garrett and Jason.

A Sprinkle of FUN from Tammy...

:An archaeologist is best husband a woman can have: the older she gets, the more interested he is in her."
-- Agatha Christie

Susan's Story
Susan Thomas

I was born to be a nurse. Since I was 5 years old I wanted to be a nurse. I can actually recall the time when I realized that my ultimate goal was to be a nurse. That dream was never questioned and has never faltered as I proceeded through life's journey. As a teenager I volunteered as a "Candy Striper". I also volunteered at a local hospital, worked as a nurse's assistant during school and found my soul at rest caring for others. Reaching out and making others feel better about themselves during a difficult time has been my motto - forever.

I have always been a patient advocate for others going above and beyond to get answers and results for the patients and families I cared for. I honor my profession and I have had a wonderful career as a nurse focusing in oncology that included home care, hospice care and patient education. At Grace Hospital, in Detroit, I taught the American Cancer Society "I Can Cope" class and brought people together to talk about their diagnosis and treatment issues. My years of clinical experience form a foundation for my service to clients today. I am most comfortable providing service – it's in my blood. I have been the caregiver and cared for both of my parents as they aged, being their voice and advocate for years.

I was diagnosed in 1992 and elected to have a mastectomy and full course of chemotherapy. It was a strange experience finding myself on the other side of the fence. I had been working with cancer patients my entire career. I quickly discovered the trials experienced with the initial diagnosis and ensuing treatment. My entire family was engaged and we all worked together to get through this period.

I wasn't going to let cancer control me. I used a hypnotherapist to help me through chemotherapy. As a practicing Oncology Nurse Clinician I was trying to figure out what my new normal was going to be. I was bald, had purchased a wig that didn't fit. I almost lost it at Disney World. Thanks to my daughter's quick reaction when she put her hand on my wig it was not lost. I read a quote by Henry Ford "Whether You Think You Can or You Can't, You're Right." My husband encouraged me to design a hat that will be comfortable and stylish on a bald head. After that my mission and destiny were defined. I contacted a local designer to create hats for me to wear. I received so many positive comments my husband said "let's talk to women's boutiques and salons to see if they would be interested in providing hats for women who have experienced cancer treatment and lost their hair." We wound up selling a growing list of products to more than 800 retail stores nationwide. In fact, we also had retail boutiques in Scotland, England, and even in Singapore. We expanded, opened a retail shop, created a Web site to offer products to women sharing the same experience.

I know what it's like to go through chemo and lose my hair – I lived it. As an Oncology Nurse I never realized what patients experienced with hair loss. I think that's what makes Susan's Special Needs so unique. We look at ourselves providing solutions to women who are undergoing medical treatment. Just because you have been affected by cancer doesn't mean you shouldn't feel beautiful.

At Susan's Special Needs we carry an ever growing range of products including more than 2,000 wigs, turbans, hats, scarves, mastectomy bras and lingerie to fit many different breast forms; swimsuits with mastectomy pockets, pajamas, tank tops and loungewear for women experiencing hot flashes; and a line of skin care products designed for those during radiation treatment and chemotherapy.

We develop an action plan for clients to help them better understand they are not alone and have products available to meet their needs on their journey. We present women with options and then let them decide what's best for them. Our goal is to help make this a positive experience. In fact, one of the most important services we provide is to find the right wig for women who have lost their hair. Traditional fashion wigs won't hold up under daily use. We carry the best wigs designed and manufactured from around the globe. We take great care to find the right color and style, then custom tailor the wigs for each client. It's a lot like going to the beauty salon. Women may be self-conscious at first, but it quickly turns into a very positive, enjoyable experience for them.

A big part of making it enjoyable is giving our clients privacy and being there to comfort and encourage them. There's a lot of hugging and counseling in our interaction with our clients.

Hair loss evokes different emotions in women. It makes the whole cancer experience real for them, and that's when the fear comes in. But once they see how beautiful they look, they breathe a sigh of relief. We just put a smile on their face and get them to laugh.

My true goal at Susan's Special Needs is to give women a boost of confidence and a more positive outlook on life. Because I've been through it all myself, I think women look at me and say, 'If she can do it, I can do it.' It's so rewarding to make a difference in the journey of these people.

I never would have dreamed that combining my oncology nursing experience with my breast cancer experience at Susan's Special Needs would have been so fulfilling providing a new life balance and the opportunity to meet so many beautiful people.

For more information about Susan and her business, please check out her website at: www.susansspecialneeds.com

Insects and Animals
Jim Tudor
In Loving Memory of Coleen Tudor

On a cold winter night in February I was abruptly snatched from deep in the heart of dreamland and brought back to reality by the scream of my wife. " What is the matter?" I exclaimed. She replied, "Something bit me". I said, "You must have had a nightmare". She said. "No, something bit me", as she jumped up and raced to the bathroom to look at the wound under a bright light.

A few seconds later she emerged and said "Something bit me here on the left breast". Then she snapped on the light and ripped the blanket off a startled husband. She said, "Get up, we have to find what bit me", as she proceeded to remove the sheets and pillow cases. A thorough search of the bed, underneath it, and surrounding areas but the biting monster in the night had escaped unharmed.

Coleen went back into the bathroom and applied antiseptic to the wound while I put the bedroom back together and we went back to sleep. The morning light revealed a small red mark that was slightly itchy but seemed to be nothing to worry about. A couple of weeks passed but the red mark did not. A couple of more weeks passed and the red mark had started to grow. By this time Coleen had become a little worried and made an appointment with the doctor. The physician's assistant examined the afflicted area and said it was nothing to worry about, just a minor reaction to either the spider's venom or perhaps a slight infection. She prescribed an antibiotic and said, "That should take care of it in a week or so, if not call back and I'll renew the prescription."

Two weeks passed and the red mark was still growing. Another round of antibiotics did not help. By this time Coleen was becoming quite concerned. The red mark was now about the size of a silver dollar and very sensitive. Coleen scheduled another appointment and went to see the doctor again. This time she asked the physician's assistant, "Do you think I could have breast cancer?" The lady said, "You have an infection that is not responding to the antibiotic. I will prescribe a different one. Spider bites do not cause cancer. If you do not respond to the new prescription in a week call and I will try another".

The new prescription had no effect nor did the one that followed. This time when Coleen scheduled an appointment she insisted on seeing the doctor, not the assistant. The doctor examined the area and told Coleen not to worry and there was no reason to check for cancer, it was just an infection and she prescribed more antibiotics. The new antibiotics had no effect. Four more weeks had passed and by this time the breast had become swollen and painful. The two small fang marks were now quite prominent and discharging a fluid. The pain was so great that Coleen pricked the wound. A large amount of fluid came spurting out. Coleen called the doctor and demanded that a mammogram be scheduled. She reminded the doctor that she was fifty three and had never had a mammogram. The doctor reminded Coleen that she did not usually order mammograms for ladies under fifty-five unless there was a history of problems in the family. She once again assured Coleen there was no reason to worry about breast cancer because spider bites do not cause cancer.

More antibiotics were prescribed and a mammogram was ordered. The situation worsened as we waited for the test. In the meantime, Spring had arrived. Coleen and I loved to sit on the patio enjoying the beauty of our large pear tree in bloom. One evening after dinner I said. "Let's go out and sit on the patio for a while". Coleen replied, "I can't, the bees won't leave me alone. I was out this afternoon and they came swarming after me. I don't want to get stung." I went out to sit on the patio. After a short while Coleen came out and sure enough the bees left the blossoms to swarm around her. I teased her saying, "The bees like you because you are so sweet".

The next evening after dinner I suggested that we go out and sit on the swing as it was quite a distance from the pear tree and I felt Coleen would not attract the bees from there. She said, "I can't, Bear will attack me". Bear was a very affectionate cat who loved to be petted all the time. "Why do you say that", I asked. The only thing Bear ever does is occasionally jump up on the swing to get attention. He's your buddy! "Twice today I went out to sit on the swing and Bear attacked me", she replied. "The first time Bear was sitting on the swing next to me. I was petting him when all of a sudden he tried to bite me on the breast. I tossed him off but he went around the back of the swing and jumped up on the back of it and tried to scratch my breast. I chased him off, but about five minutes later he came back. He sat and looked at me for a few minutes then he jumped on my chest and tried to bite my breast again. Thankfully I wasn't hurt but I'm not going to take any more chances I have enough problems without having to deal with bites or scratches."

I went out to sit on the swing and found Bear to be his usual affectionate self. I wondered why he acted the way he had earlier in the day. The following week the mammogram was performed. The results were no signs of lumps or other abnormalities. Coleen and I were greatly relieved. She finished taking the latest round of antibiotics but the condition persisted. We were about to call the doctor again when Coleen received a phone call. Another doctor had taken a look at Coleen's mammogram and discovered a cloudy looking area. He wanted another mammogram taken. A few days later the mammogram had been taken and the results came back. The doctor was not sure what the test revealed but as a precautionary measure he wanted a biopsy performed on the spot in question.

The biopsy was performed. The results were Coleen's worst nightmare come true. She did indeed have cancer. The surgeon who performed the biopsy wanted to schedule surgery about a month later. However, Coleen was quite unsatisfied with the treatment our rural health care system had been providing. She called Magee Women's Hospital in Pittsburgh for an appointment. A surgeon was assigned and she went to see him two days later.

The surgeon met with us and informed Coleen he could operate four days later. Coleen said, "Can't I think about this for another week or so?" The surgeon replied, "This is an emergency situation. The tumor has doubled in size in the two weeks between the biopsy and today. I will be away for the next four weeks. If you wait until I return there will be no hope of survival." The surgery was performed successfully. Thankfully she was given two more years before the cancer returned and metastasized cutting her life short.

My message to those who read this is that nature sees far more accurately than doctors and their fancy machines. If you or a loved one suddenly attracts insects and animals pay attention, dogs and cats can smell cancer long before it is visible on tests. Your pets love you. When they attempt to scratch or bite you they are attacking the tumor to protect you from it.

Jim lives in the heart of The Magic Forest area of Western PA. Jim is a business coach who works with organizations that want their managers to become outstanding leaders. You can visit Jim's site at: www.thekingofleaders.com.

A Sprinkle of FUN from Tammy...

Women are always beautiful. -- Ville Valo

Linked by Pink
Michelle Wagner

Hearing you have a cancer diagnosis once is scary enough, but hearing it again seven years later really makes you wonder if it's going to, ultimately, get the best of you. I was first diagnosed in February 2003 with Stage 0-DCIS Breast Cancer. I had only been working at Edinboro University for 3 months when I got the news and, although it was shocking, the prognosis was good. We had "caught it early" and 8 months and four surgeries later I was deemed "cancer free!" That, I thought, was the end of my own personal battle with cancer.

Then, six months into my new job at Gannon University and almost seven years to the day, my doctor called my husband, Shane, and I into his office on February 8th. I had been experiencing pain in my left hip and, although I felt like a hypochondriac, once you've had a cancer diagnosis there's always this little voice inside your head that whispers, "What if?" So, listen to your body! An abnormal x-ray led to an abnormal bone scan which finally led to a bone biopsy that confirmed the worst. Breast cancer cells were now in the bone of my left hip, sternum and thoracic spine. Looks like I'll be retiring at Gannon, because with this kind of a track record with new jobs, my husband says I'm not allowed to change jobs ever again! So, I underwent 2 more surgeries in March and started treatments every 3 weeks which will continue for at least a year.

I'm not alone in this journey though, which is both good and bad. Friends have found themselves in the same boat as me; Matt, Pat, Lori, Ted, Barb, Lisa, Kim, Chrissy and all the Linked by Pink ladies. Hopefully, together, we'll all be able to help one another successfully navigate through this. I know I've charted my "thumb line" and set my sights on the horizon and the point at which I've put this cancer thing in my wake once again and hope everyone else can do the same. Grandpa Alex, Grandpa Butch, D.J., Becky, Coach Corbett, Renae, Brian, Uncle Jerry and Sharon; I love and miss you all and think of you often as I sail these waters.

353

I certainly don't claim to understand this disease or why it keeps claiming our best and our brightest, but it's the memories of those who have lost their battle, along with the rest of my family and friends who are still with me, that make it possible for me to keep fighting and make sticking around for as long as I can so worthwhile. There's no way I'm going to let this thing get the best of me! So, anytime anything but positive thoughts enter my mind, I simply remind myself of the "battle cry" given to me the day after my Uncle Jerry's funeral when my brother, Michael, gathered us all together to pray. "I believe I have received my healing!" And I pray others receive theirs as well.

Michelle lives in McKean, PA with her husband, Shane, his son, Cody and their family pets, Dakota, Daisy and Moses. She is the Assistant Director of Recreation and Wellness at Gannon University's Carneval Athletic Pavilion in Erie, PA and is an Adjunct Lecturer in the Sport and Exercise Science Program there as well. She enjoys sailing, outdoor activities, their new pool and newly renovated home and spending time with family and friends.

I Believe Cancer Sucks...
Becky Sharp Ward

Cancer may suck but the bottom line is: cancer saved my life. I listen to women tell their stories; and I have lived their pain.

A few years before my diagnosis, I struggled through a painful divorce. The divorce was a surprise to me. I was content, happy in my life, even satisfied. When the facts of my ex husband's other life came to my attention, I was devastated. The pain was unbearable. Others could see my pain, but no one could help me as I spiraled through the mental anguish I called my life. I found comfort with medication, alcohol and depression. I found myself in and out of mental hospitals. I had quit life.

I was in the process of climbing out of my pit of self pity when my doctor spoke those words no one wants to hear – Cancer. The previous two years of my life had been a mess, and now this? I had a fleeting fear of falling back into the hole of despair I had been in before. I decided this time was going to be different. I asked for help; something that had been hard for me to do during my divorce. But fortunately, I learn from my mistakes. And boy, was I happy I did! As I bravely told my friends of my diagnosis, I was offered all kinds of HELP; really great help. People offered stories of their family and friends who were survivors; people called to offer support, my family circled around me again; I found friends I didn't even know I had! And I heard the word "survivor" over and over.

I wasn't really familiar with the term SURVIVOR.

I was lucky to connect with an advocacy group (not really a support group) called PINK (Power IN Knowledge). Each month when the group gathered, there was a custom at the beginning of the meeting, to tell everyone how long you've been a survivor. My first night, when it was my turn, with uncertainty I said "I don't really know if I'm a survivor since I was just diagnosed." Well, the room erupted with laughter and enlightenment! "You are a survivor from the day you are diagnosed!" Just the ice breaker I needed- I decided at that moment that I was in for the fight, and I was blessed that I had found others to help me with my fight!

My family was very worried about my physical and mental health. They had spent many months with me nursing my heart, mind and spirit through the divorce process. And what I discovered was this was the time for me to lean on them and let them help me build MY strength.

Armed with information from my wonderful surgeon, I moved forward with such great confidence in my own decisions. When the diagnosis indicated that I needed a mastectomy followed by chemo, I shed a tear, and mourned the change my body was going to experience. But I felt empowered that finally, I was in charge of my life and my decisions were my own.

So why am I so grateful for the cancer that could have killed me? Because it brought me back to ME. I was reminded that I was important, people did care. I needed to get better not only physically but mentally because I was a MOM, a CHILD, a SISTER, an AUNT and a FRIEND to many. I just couldn't QUIT like I did before. I could not let the people who supported me through my divorce down again.

Cancer made me fight. It did not beat me. Maybe I was looking for the fight I never got through the divorce process. And just maybe I was happy to put my energy into a fight worth fighting for. Breast cancer was not going to win.

When I asked a question, my surgeon, plastic surgeon or oncologist, gave me an honest, sincere answer. It was not always the answer I may have been looking for, but I was finally getting heart felt honesty and integrity from someone I wanted to trust. My doctors listened to me cry, supported my choices, and treated me with respect. For this, I will always love them.

I have moved on with my life. I live in a wonderful supportive community surrounded by my friends and family. Though my children are still working through the pains of divorce, the pain of watching their mother suffer through a cancer diagnosis is over. We have healed.

Every once in a while I get a text message from one of my boys, now away in college. It may just be a silly text about the weather but it reminds me I am loved. And that's all we want. To be loved.

So if you have been faced with the Big C, please only despair for a minute. There is a light at the end of the tunnel. Let your friends and family wrap their arms around you and hold you up. Trust me, you will need it. And in the end, when you are still around to thank them with a big smile, do so. Don't hesitate. Because love is the only thing that really keeps us humans going, and in this day and age, love can go a long way.

Good luck and God Bless, Becky

Becky lives in Dallastown, PA with her 2 college age sons, Miss Puddy Cat and 2 aquatic turtles. She sells kitchen cabinets for a living but would rather work in her garden. You can contact her at caseddie@comcast.net.

A Sprinkle of FUN from Tammy...

"I don't have false teeth. Do you think I'd buy teeth like these?"
-- Carol Burnett

Now, I Am Enjoying Retirement!
Colleen Weaver

My story actually begins in June, 2007 which is the date I retired from 34 years of service with the Commonwealth of PA. In July I had my typical annual mammogram and everything was fine. By October of 2007 I felt a lump in my right breast and through several tests, it was confirmed, I had Stage 2 Breast Cancer. Needless to say, this was not my idea of the way to start retirement.

I struggled with the idea of not having any surgery, chemo and/or radiation because my children were on their own and my husband can be very self sufficient so why put myself through this? What I didn't know at the time is that this is a very common emotional roller coaster for women faced with breast cancer.

One thing I could always count on through my journey was the support from God, all my friends, family and people I never met even when I wasn't so sure I could or wanted to make it myself.

I also learned to count the small blessings and look carefully because they were there. Some of the blessings I found along the way include:

- Finding out the day after my diagnosis that I was going to be a grandma for the first time - THIS WAS A HUGE BLESSING AND SURELY A LIGHT AT THE END OF MY TUNNEL.

- Keeping my hair until after the funeral of my father-in-law. It fell out the day after he was buried.

- Not having to shave my legs and armpits and subsequent savings on shampoo, conditioner and razor blades.

- One thing I learned which may help other survivors is how I am handling "Chemo Brain." I found that taking zumba and tap lessons, has significantly helped my memory and concentration. I

358

seem to be able to concentrate better on the task at hand rather than having the "fog affect" that chemotherapy can sometimes produce.

- The arrival of meals when I didn't ask for them but they came at a time most needed and appreciated.

- Keeping a sense of humor even when things looked the bleakest. For example, the day when I was in such a hurry to put a casserole in the oven so I could get to my first Cancer Support Group Meeting. The reason I was in such a hurry is that I had just had my first radiation treatment appointment with the Dr. and was informed that once everything was set up, I would need 6 weeks and it wouldn't start until 2 weeks after I had planned because I wanted to be done by the time my granddaughter was to be born on June 19.

Anyway after opening the pre-heated oven door, I burnt the bangs on my wig. While I was crying, I decided I was still going to make this meeting and proceeded to curl my eyelashes. It was as if God said, "You want something to cry about, I'll give you something to cry about" and at that moment, I accidently pulled out the last three eyelashes I had. This made me laugh and I still made it to the meeting.

- Getting funny e-mails from people during my darkest moments.

- Belonging to a wonderful sisterhood called "Breast Cancer Survivors."

This July will mark 3 years since my last cancer treatment and I am proud to say I am cancer free and now have two grandchildren who I love to pieces. The one thing I wish I would have known before going through all this is that even when you have completed all the treatments, it takes a good year or longer until you actually feel like yourself again.

I am now enjoying my retirement and have the energy back to do the things I want.

Colleen Weaver is married and originally from Lansing, MI and now living in Palmyra, PA. She has two grown children and two grandchildren who are the light of her life. She can be reached at Nuts4MI@msn.com.

A Sprinkle of FUN from Tammy...

"The heyday of woman's life is the shady side of fifty."
-- Elizabeth Cady Stanton

One Cool Woman
Haralee Weintraub

After the breast cancer treatments threw me into menopause with drenching night sweats I knew there were many women like me, not getting a good night sleep. For oncologists the protocol is all about eliminating the cancer, but for the patient it is about a quality of life. I chose to help women like myself going through this experience to get a more comfortable night sleep and improve their quality of life. I started my own company of wicking sleepwear, Haralee.Com with the mission to make 'Cool Garments for Hot Women'.

For my models I use real women who are friends or friends of friends, or daughters or grand daughters who have had breast cancer, or been touched first hand by cancer. I have women asking to model for me now because they want to show that life can continue after cancer. Initially I only used age appropriate women, women who would be menopausal age, but I had younger women wanting to model who were cancer survivors. I now include women in a wide range of ages. My goal is to show that breast cancer has no one claim to an age group or ethnicity, but that all women can still look beautiful living with cancer. I design all our styles with the breast cancer survivor in mind. We don't use any buttons or fancy do-dads that may irritate sensitive skin from surgeries or radiation. All the fabrics I pick out, I seek a soft feel that will be next to sensitive skin.

Any woman who is diagnosed with cancer has to become her own health advocate. She has to evaluate all the information the doctors are giving her and make her own decisions. One of the decisions after my cancer treatments I made after carefully looking at my career path was to leave my corporate job and become an entrepreneur. Breast cancer gave me the courage to make a career change. After looking at a life threatening diagnosis, starting my own business seemed easy!

In a millions years I never thought a breast cancer diagnosis would lead to becoming an entrepreneur. I never thought my business would not be successful because I knew I was helping other women get a better night sleep.

Because I want my customers to feel good about their purchase on every level, and breast cancer has had such a profound impact on my life, I donate a percentage of every sale to breast cancer research. We are a company with a lot of heart, a lot of soul, and a little bit too much sweat. My primary care physician and my oncologist have been supportive fans of my business and refer patients expressing night sweat issues to my web site.

Tammy asked me to respond to a few questions:

One of the things I learned from my experience with breast cancer and in starting my own company is courage and taking risks. I went in for a routine physical and mammogram, feeling healthy and told I was very ill. I didn't feel sick until the chemo treatments made me sick. Facing recovery from surgeries, chemo, radiation and my own mortality gave me the courage to really look at my career and work life. I questioned my legacy. I wanted to give back and help other women so I started my own company.

I use vibrant colors for my sleepwear because I know when I was going through treatments and the following year, I wanted happy colors around me. I even bought a bright yellow car.

My advice to other women is to take another person with you to all appointments and a recorder. Don't think you will be the unusual person who has no side effects, who will bounce back in a week, who can ignore your treatments. If you do this you are setting yourself up for disappointment and a pocket full of anxiety. Give yourself a break and ask for help from friends and family on daily household chores like cleaning, laundry, cooking, and meal preparation.

I also advise other women to be prepared for stupid things people will say. Many people don't know what to say so they will tell you some story trying to connect and encourage but it can come across having the opposite effect. Shield yourself from the negative toxic people who can be cancer wannabes, or into big dramas. Although they may want to help you there usually are others that have no other agendas than to be helpful.

The loss of hair happens over the whole body. What this means is no nose hairs. Never knew their purpose before but I had a drippy nose for 4 months during the cold months of the year. I had some pretty hankies and now when I know someone is going through chemo treatments, I give hankies. Eyebrows define a face well and can be drawn with cosmetics. The problem I had was all the hot flashes made me sweaty and often I would catch myself with a brow melting and heading south down my cheek! Another use for a hanky, wipe and re-apply.

I asked my oncologist what I could do to help with my treatments so I would have an active part in fighting the disease and recovery. He suggested some alternative treatments along with the conventional treatments. I started acupuncture twice a week the same week I started chemo. I think it helped with my side effects but it also helped me feel proactive in my care. My oncologist also suggested some clinical trials. To date I have participated in six clinical trails. This participation makes me feel that I am giving back and paying it forward.

Sincerely Cool,
Haralee Weintraub

Haralee is the CEO of Haralee.Com Sleepwear, Cool Garments for Hot Women. You can reach her at: www.haralee.com or haralee@haralee.com

My Experience with the "Pink Ribbon Story" Project
Diane Weller

Interviewing breast cancer survivors and their families and writing their stories, has been humbling and personally rewarding. Hearing personal accounts of pain, suffering, extreme fear, and the battle to maintain normalcy in a world turned upside-down reminds me to always count my blessings and to reach out to others through prayer and through other forms of help.

For some, it was difficult to begin their story – they were not sure what to say. Discovering my ability to have strangers completely open up to me and share very personal experiences and thoughts was a reward not anticipated going into this project. As one caregiver husband I spoke to said, "I never sat down and formulated my thoughts about it". It is my hope that by talking with this individual in a sensitive and caring way, he has felt a sense of freedom from the difficult experience he has endured and can talk about it more freely from this day on.

Hearing and writing about these stories causes me to think about the incredible strength and resiliency of women. Whether dealing with a bald head or the removal of one's breasts, in a society where neither is a cultural norm, and enduring the extreme after pain of breast removal, these women serve as a source of inspiration to never give up on whatever challenge(s) we are presented.

There is always someone out there dealing with a life challenge greater than our own. I encourage you to reach out a helping hand.

--Diane Weller
"Ring the bells that still can ring, forget your perfect offering. There is a crack in everything; that's how the light gets in." ~ lyrics from Leonard Cohen's Anthem

Diane Weller is a proud mother of two beautiful, successful daughters, the wife of a selfless and supportive husband, and an independent woman. In her dual career as parent and IT professional, Diane's leadership journey has given her joy in helping others develop through her supervising, mentoring, and peer coaching. Diane is looking forward to new and exciting personal and professional accomplishments in the years ahead.

A Sprinkle of FUN from Tammy...

"In politics, if you want anything said, ask a man - if you want anything done, ask a woman."

-- Margaret Thatcher

A Life Change for the Better
Nancy White

I was diagnosed with Stage II breast cancer at the age of 48. I had never had a mammogram before but I had a nagging feeling that I should have one done. Sure enough I got a call that I needed to come back for another mammogram because there was something abnormal.

I ended up with invasive lobular Aden carcinoma that had spread to one of my lymph nodes. Thank God I listened to that voice in my head and had that mammogram done. I had just had a physical exam three months before my mammogram and my doctor didn't feel any lumps, nor did I or my breast surgeon.

It turns out that I had three tumors in my breast and needed to have a mastectomy. I underwent eight rounds of chemotherapy and six weeks of radiation therapy and now almost two and a half years later I am doing very well.

I am grateful to have been through this experience. I have learned that I am a lot stronger than I thought I was. My marriage is stronger than it was before. My faith in God has grown. I have always been very shy but had the honor of speaking, along with my breast surgeon, at a press conference about the importance of women under the age of 50 having mammograms when the recommendations were changed two years ago. Our church has started a support group for cancer patients, survivors and their caregivers and my husband and I are very involved with this group.

Breast cancer has changed my life forever but I believe it changed it for the better.

Nancy lives in Lewisburg, PA with her husband of 31 years James. They have one son, Stephen. She works as the Medical Records Director at RiverWoods in Lewisburg, PA.

One Step at a Time
Diana Whisler

I am a 4 time cancer survivor, with three being breast cancer related.

I was in bed one night in August of 1999 (divorced only one year and 44 years old) and felt an unusual tingling going down my left arm. I started feeling around and found a lump. The next morning I called my ob-gyn and made an appointment. He examined me and said it was nothing, just go home and have a glass of wine and forget about it. I insisted on a biopsy. He sent me to a local surgeon and what a nightmare experience that was.

The surgeon stuck a huge needle in my breast and jiggled it around until he thought he had what he needed. He told me if it comes back as cancer he will have me back to his office and will remove it with a local anesthesia and then I can go home. I wouldn't need a driver as I will be able to drive myself. I was horrified. I thought about this for several weeks and then it was time to go back for the results.

I decided to have a consult with my family doctor and told him what the surgeon said. He called for my results and it WAS cancer. Of course I cried and cried. He then referred me to a breast cancer specialist in York, PA. I told the doctor that I wanted to save my breast so he did a sentinel node biopsy and lumpectomy. I had one node positive and I opted not to take chemo so I went to the radiation doctor who reviewed my test results and sent me back to the surgeon to get more of a clear margin around the original lump that was removed.

My surgeon was furious that I opted out of chemo and said he would personally take me to John Hopkins for a second opinion as he thought I was too young to refuse chemo and the chances of survival would be better with chemo. I had a second surgery and still not clear margins. I told my surgeon to take the breast off but he asked for one last chance so into surgery we went again. This was followed by four rounds of chemotherapy and six weeks of radiation.

367

After my first round of chemotherapy I was sitting at breakfast with my new friend and he said that he wanted to take me to Florida after I was done with treatment as I had never been there. I told him that I did not want to go to Florida after I was bald so the next day at 9 AM I was on a plane! We were there for a week and the day we came back my hair started to fall out!

I was in remission until November of 2009 when I went in for a routine exam and my surgeon had found that my supraclavicular node was enlarged. After a biopsy it was found that the breast cancer had spread to the lymph nodes in my neck. Further tests also proved that I had medullary thyroid cancer. Another operation and chemotherapy and three weeks of radiation when I found out that my now husband had contracted a staph infection from the hospital when he went in for kidney stones. He was within hours of dying so I had to stop my radiation treatments to take care of him.

I was in remission again until January of 2011 when it was discovered that the breast cancer was now in the lymph nodes under my breast bone. I am now on Xeloda chemotherapy pills with a co-payment of $757.00 every three weeks. I looked everywhere for help but because I have a full time job, I make too much money! No one asks how many bills you have to pay! I have finally gotten help from Genetech, the makers of Xeloda. They said they will help with up to 80% of the co-pay.

The hardest part in the beginning of my journey was telling my daughter who was a sophomore in high school in 1999. She decided to hold a walk for breast cancer as her senior graduation project! She raised $2000 for the PA BREAST CANCER COALITION. We have walked in two Susan G Komen 3 day walks together (2008 & 2009). She has participated in the Global Race For The Cure in Washington, DC. and she also participated this last November in another 3-day walk with her sister-in-law. We have a team called the "Pink Ribbon Ladies" that consists of my daughter, daughter-in-law, son and several of their close friends, and have we raised over $36,000 for breast cancer research with the monies going to the American Cancer Society, Susan G Komen and our local "Pink Out" fund.

Diana lives in Abbottstown, PA with her husband of 7 years, Fred. They have 2 cats and between them, they have 5 grown children and 7 grandchildren. She manages the office at ADESA PA auto auction. She loves gardening as it keeps her mind off of the cancer! Her email is diana.whisler@yahoo.com.

A Sprinkle of FUN from Tammy…

"I used to be Snow White, but I drifted."

-- Mae West

Fighting the Fight for Hope
Rhonda Wolford

June 3, 2005 is a day that changed my life - - a diagnosis which began a journey of many ups and downs, but also a journey that has tested my faith, and brought my family together closer than ever. I have found strength and courage inside myself that I never knew existed. After 6 weeks of testing an area that my doctor felt was only "dense breast tissue" my diagnosis came. I was only 35 years old and my daughters were ages 13 and 10. I was so scared that I wasn't going to be here to see them grow up. I thank God that I did some research about breast cancer symptoms and pushed for further testing because my story today could be much different. It is SO important to be proactive about your health. You need to be your own advocate.

The first few weeks after my diagnosis were very difficult. Our family had always been very active with the Shippensburg Relay for Life and we were only a week away from the 2005 Relay weekend. I wasn't sure I could handle being there. The only thing I wanted to do at that point was hide under the covers - - but I knew deep down that I HAD to go ~ I HAD to begin my battle and our family worked too hard all year and I didn't want them to miss the event. I had my long hair cut that day for wigs for kids ~ I hadn't planned it ahead of time, but watching my niece have hers cut that day, I just felt it was the right thing to do. Looking back, that was my first step to battle this monster we call Cancer. While walking in the survivor lap with my husband Kevin and our two daughters, Jessica and Emily, at my side, our ACS rep at that time, Amy, held up a purple "SURVIVOR" t-shirt so that I could read the word "SURVIVOR"!!!! I will never forget how that made me feel ~ it gave me such HOPE that I COULD get through the surgeries and treatments ahead of me, and that life would go on, and that I could be a SURVIVOR.

My treatment began with 8 rounds of chemotherapy. After chemo came a double mastectomy (which was my personal choice), followed by 28 radiation treatments. The medical team that was involved with my treatment were amazing and caring people and the support I received from my family, friends, church family, minister, co-workers, my employer, and people I don't even know has been phenomenal!   Cancer is a horrible disease, but when it strikes, it is incredible how people come together and offer support. The power of prayer is so awesome ~ I truly believe the prayers of many people gave me the strength and courage to endure all I had to face. I never got sick from the chemo – what a blessing! I was able to continue to work during treatments since I tolerated the chemo so well, and what a blessing that was ~ it kept me busy and made the time go by much quicker. My husband was my rock. He would always encourage me and remind me that there would be brighter days ahead. I worried how my daughters would be affected, but I truly believe it has left a positive impact on their lives. I am so proud of their drive to be involved and raise money for the ACS. Our youngest daughter, Emily, has expressed the desire to pursue a career in the medical field.   With each surgery she became an active caregiver, wanting to learn and help in any way she could. On my last day of chemo I came home to my own "flower shop".   My family arranged for me to be showered with flowers as a celebration of my last chemo treatment! I received 76 flower arrangements that day! What an unforgettable moment!

As I celebrated a year of survivorship I elected to have reconstruction surgery, which involved many surgeries over a few months until completed. I also elected to have genetic testing. I wanted to know if I developed breast cancer due to a mutation so that my daughters would have that important piece of information. I tested negative, which means they will not need to be tested.

After years of raising money for the American Cancer Society, never would I have imagined my name being read at the luminary ceremony, but we deal with what has been put in front of us. It's not easy, but you have to put one foot in front of the other and take one day at a time. I will never completely understand the Lord's plan for my life, I just know whatever path He leads me on,

He will be there every step of the way. He has carried me through the darkest times and has been so faithful.

Cancer has now affected my life directly and I have made the commitment to keep fighting harder for those who cannot fight, and to honor and celebrate those who have battled it. Because of my diagnosis, my life has changed. It has lit a fire in me to become more involved with Relay and to spread the word about my story in the hopes that it will help others become more proactive about their health, to get regular screenings, and to talk about their concerns with their doctors. No one ever wants to hear they have a diagnosis of cancer, but early detection is the key. We never know what the future holds, we can only live for today and be grateful for each day we are given. As I celebrate my 6-year survivorship at the 2011 Relay for Life in a few weeks, I will continue to fight the fight in the hopes that we will one day reach our ultimate goal ~ a cure to cancer!!

Rhonda lives in Shippensburg, PA with her wonderful family, consisting of her husband Kevin, two daughters Jessica and Emily, and 2 dogs and 3 cats. She works at a law office in Shippensburg and continues to co-chair the Shippensburg Relay for Life as her way of "fighting back" against cancer in the hopes of a cure to cancer someday. She can be reached at wolford4@comcast.net. "Life isn't about waiting for the storm to pass... it's learning how to dance in the rain"

Thank you!
Cheri Woll

Thank you for letting me into your life.

Thank you for opening up to me when you were so overwhelmed and scared.

Thank you for being so honest and showing me your raw emotions.

Thank you for letting me get to know you and your family.

Thank you for not being afraid to talk about your cancer when I might have been.

Thank you for allowing me to observe as you got your mammogram, ultrasound, biopsy, CT sim, or radiation treatment.

Thank you for allowing me to accompany you from the Breast Care Center to the hospital after your needle localization.

Thank you for allowing me to stay with you during your doctor's visit.

Thank you for allowing me to sit with you while chemo dripped into your arm.

Thank you for letting me visit with you in the Radiation Oncology department or the inpatient unit.

Thank you for trusting me enough to call me when you had a question or concern.

Thank you for letting me know when things were going well and when someone or something had let you down.

Thank you for attending the Breast Cancer Support Group and sharing your story with others.

Thank you for letting me enter your circle of support - the Cancer Survivor's Association Support Group.

Thank you for your dedication to Pink Zone.

Thank you for all that you have taught me in my first few months as the Oncology Nurse Navigator at Mount Nittany Medical Center.

And thank you for all that you will continue to teach me and share with me. I am honored to walk with you on this journey of survivorship.

Many, many thanks!!!

Cheri lives in Boalsburg, PA with her husband Ken, her son Joey (20), and her daughter Rachel (17). Their household is run by their 22 pound cat, Toby and their 7 pound dog, Trixie. Cheri has been a Registered Nurse for over 25 years and is the Oncology Nurse Navigator at Mount Nittany Medical Center. She can be reached at 231-7005 or cwoll@mountnittany.org.

Lifted by the Courage
Linda Young

I am excited to be part of Tammy's editing team again for her latest insightful book. I met Tammy years ago through Toastmasters and we've been friends ever since.

Reading these inspirational and hopeful stories has changed my life. I have lost some wonderful friends to this disease, and these stories give me hope that the battle can be won.

As my father dies from lung cancer, I am lifted up by the courage of the women, and men, of the Pink Ribbon Stories. This book is sure to be a must-read for anyone connected to the breast cancer experience.

Linda lives in Pittsburgh and is a long-time Toastmaster. She is a past marathoner and the mother of two grown children. Her three grandsons keep her lively! She spends spare time reading and editing books for her friends!

One More Round with the Big "C"
Eileen "Lee" Zoll

One can just imagine my consternation when a Gynecologist informed me that I had a malignant growth on my left breast. Over the previous twenty years I had survived three malignant melanomas that had spread to the lymph nodes. "Why me?" I asked God. "Well, why not you?"....He seemed to say. "Okay, I'll deal with it but do I have a mastectomy or should I go with one of the other options??"

For me, with my past history, I rationalized that there really was not a choice - if you have gangrene in your finger, you have it cut off. So 'Good Bye" left "boob." Due to the fact that we had moved, I needed to search for a new Oncologist. Fortunately, I found a very reputable team in the Andrews/Patel group of Camp Hill, PA and was treated like an individual with thoughts and feelings rather than "patient number ten in room two.."

As before, the lymph nodes had been invaded and the chemotherapy treatment was rather intense. However, my husband and I developed a system: The day I cooked - we ate "out", and the next day would manage to eat the food that I had previously prepared. Reading made me sick so I turned to TV and discovered that if you missed a whole week of *As the World Turns*, they had not even started a new chapter!

We rented a cottage at the Seashore for eight months and I could look forward to the calming effect of the ocean every Friday thru Sunday. We laughed one day when my husband had to chase my wig (which we called Edna) down the boardwalk. Yes, you are right......he does spoil me and I love it!

You perhaps wonder if losing a breast had an adverse effect on our sex life. Why should it?? I lost the breast - not him! If it bothered him, he could just get over it - I was still "sexy". Eight years later, I lost my other breast, and guess what? I continue to attract his attentions, and we will be married sixty happy years in January of 2012. What else can one say but, "Thank you Lord, for the gift of life".

Eileen lives in Camp Hill, PA, and enjoys volunteering with church activities, helping raise funds for Cancer Research, and pursuing all the activities involved with having a loving, caring family. She belongs to a study club, and book club, and takes advantage of all the museums, theatrical, and musical performances that Harrisburg/New York/Philadelphia/Washington have to offer. This encourages her to explore and enjoy the world in which we live. She and her husband enjoy traveling and through their travels, they manage to find interesting antiques to sell at Golden Lane Antique Gallery in New Oxford, PA. She invites you to come and enjoy the antiques, or if you feel like getting in touch with "someone who has been there" - feel free to email her at: leezoll@aol.com.

A Sprinkle of FUN from Tammy...

"We cannot really love anybody with whom we never laugh."
-- Agnes Repplier

Notes:

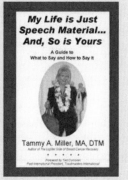

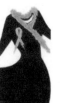
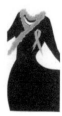
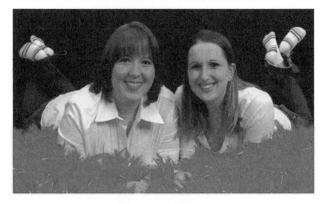

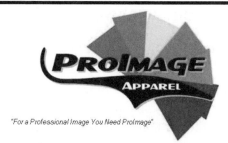
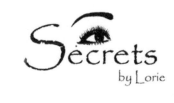

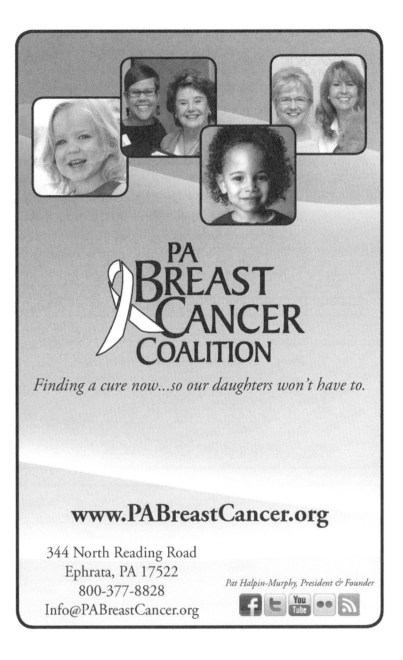

Thank you for reading
Pink Ribbon Stories:
A Celebration of Life!!

If you are interested in making a donation to
offset some of the publishing and distribution costs,
and to provide books to people who may not
otherwise receive one, please send your donations to:

Tammy A. Miller
1172 Ghaner Road
Port Matilda, PA 16870

Dear Lord,
Please use me this day
beyond my
wildest dreams!